European Paedi Advanced Life Support

C000085850

4th Edition February 2016

Reprinted in January 2017
Reprinted in May 2018

ISBN 978-1-903812-32-7

European Paediatric Advanced Life Support
4th Edition February 2016 – Reprinted in January 2017 and May 2018

Editors

Sophie Skellett
Sue Hampshire
Robert Bingham
Ian Maconochie
Sarah Mitchell

Contributors

Souhail Alouni
Dominique Biarent
Paolo Biban
Robert Bingham
Keith Brownlee
Gudrun Burda
Gerard Cheron
Fiona Clements
Karen Cooper
Mike Coren
Serena Cottrell
Fotini Danou

Jo Draaisma
Christoph Eich
Christine Fonteyne
Miguel Felix
Mojca Groselj-Grenc
Sue Hampshire
Sylvia Hunyadi-Anticevic
Ben Lakin
Torsten Lauritsen
Francis Leclerc
Anselmi Luciano
Jesus Lopez-Herce

Ian Maconochie
Ian McDougall
David Mason
Sarah Mitchell
Liz Norris
Thomas Rajka
Sam Richmond
Antonio Rodriguez-Nunez
Sheila Simpson
Ruchi Sinha
Sophie Skellett
Frederic Tits

Felicity Todd
John Trounce
Nigel Turner
Patrick Van de Voorde
Burkhard Wermter
Mark Woolcock
Mark Worrall
Jonathan Wyllie
Deborah Zeitlin
David Zideman

Acknowledgements

We thank and acknowledge the members of the ERC 2015 Guidelines Writing Group who have contributed directly or indirectly to this EPALS manual.

We thank Mark Sedge for taking the photographs for this manual and the models and their parents for giving up their time to help with these. We also thank Paul Wood for his help with the final preparation for printing.

Environmental friendly paper has been used. 15% recycled, elemental chlorine free fibre sourced from well managed forests.

Originally published by the European Resuscitation Council (2003)
Second edition (2006)
Third edition (2011)

This edition published by Resuscitation Council (UK) 2016
5th Floor, Tavistock House North, Tavistock Square, London WC1H 9HR
Tel: 020 7388 4678   Fax: 020 7383 0773   E-mail: enquiries@resus.org.uk   Website: www.resus.org.uk

Printed by: TT Litho Printers Limited
Units 3 & 5 Northpoint, Enterprise Close, Medway City Estate, Rochester, Kent ME2 4LX
Tel: 01634 845397   Email: admin@ttlitho.co.uk   Website: www.ttlitho.co.uk

The Resuscitation Council (UK) guidelines are adapted from the European Resuscitation Council guidelines and have been developed using a process accredited by The National Institute for Health and Care Excellence. The UK guidelines are consistent with the European guidelines but include minor modifications to reflect the needs of the National Health Service.

This European Paediatric Advanced Life Support (EPALS) manual is written by the Resuscitation Council (UK) EPALS Subcommittee and forms part of the resources for the Resuscitation Council (UK) EPALS course, which is delivered in accredited course centres throughout the UK.

Foreword

The European Paediatric Advanced Life Support (EPALS) provider course is a pan-European project developed under the auspices of the European Resuscitation Council. It provides training for multidisciplinary healthcare professionals in the early recognition of the child in respiratory or circulatory failure and the development of the knowledge and core skills required to prevent further deterioration towards respiratory or cardiorespiratory arrest.

The course comprises the manual, lectures, workshops, skill stations, teaching simulations and assessments. It now also encompasses many paediatric specific illnesses that those caring for children will encounter. We hope you find the manual to be informative as it contains not only information covered on the course but extra information which will be useful to your practice. We have put this additional information in a number of grey boxes in each chapter (candidates will not be tested on this information at the end of the EPALS course). Candidate interaction and participation is a key element of the face to face element of the course.

Instructors on the course teach voluntarily, giving their time and expertise without financial gain. Their enthusiasm and commitment for the subject helps to maintain the courses' high standards and ensure its availability to healthcare professionals who would be expected to apply the skills taught as part of their clinical duties.

We very much hope you enjoy the course.

Dr Sophie Skellett
Chairman, EPALS course Subcommittee,
Resuscitation Council (UK)

Glossary

- AED   Automated external defibrillator
- ABG   Arterial blood gas (needs to go above AED)
- BLS   Basic life support
- BP   Blood pressure
- CRT   Capillary refill time
- CO_2 Carbon dioxide
- CO   Cardiac output
- CPR   Cardiopulmonary resuscitation
- DNACPR   Do not attempt cardiopulmonary resuscitation
- ECG   Electrocardiogram
- FiO_2 Fraction of inspired oxygen
- HR   Heart rate
- H   Hour
- IM   Intramuscular
- IO   Intraosseous
- IV   Intravenous
- LMA   laryngeal mask airway
- Mg^{2+} Magnesium
- Min   Minute
- Na^+ Sodium
- O_2 Oxygen
- PEA   Pulseless electrical activity
- PEF   Peak expiratory flow
- PICU   Paediatric intensive care unit
- $PaCO_2$ Partial pressure of arterial carbon dioxide
- PaO_2 Partial pressure of arterial oxygen
- PEEP   Positive end expiratory pressure
- pMDI   pressurised metred dose inhaler
- K^+ Potassium
- RR   Respiratory rate
- SaO_2 Arterial oxygen saturation
- S   Second
- SGA   Supraglottic airway
- SpO_2 Peripheral oxygen saturation (pulse oximetry)
- SV   Stroke volume
- SVT   Supraventricular tachycardia
- SVR   Systemic vascular resistance
- VF   Ventricular fibrillation
- VT   Ventricular tachycardia
- pVT   pulseless ventricular tachycardia

Throughout this publication the masculine is used to denote the masculine or the feminine

Contents

Introduction to Paediatric Advanced Life Support

Contents

- **The differences between primary and secondary cardiorespiratory arrest**
- **Outcomes from respiratory and cardiorespiratory arrest in children**
- **Basic anatomy and physiology of an infant or child's airway, breathing, and circulation**
- **How differences in anatomy and physiology influence resuscitation of a seriously ill child**

Learning outcomes

To enable you to:

- **Understand how aetiologies of cardiorespiratory arrest in children differ from those in adults**
- **Discuss probable outcomes of primary and secondary cardiorespiratory arrest**
- **Describe why specific anatomical and physiological characteristics of infants and young children influence their clinical management**

Aetiologies of cardiorespiratory arrest

The aetiology of cardiorespiratory arrest in children differs from adults. This is due to anatomical, physiological and pathological differences, which alter throughout childhood.

Primary cardiorespiratory arrest is a sudden acute event, which occurs without warning. It is commonly due to a cardiac arrhythmia reflecting intrinsic heart disease. Successful outcome is generally dependent on rapid defibrillation, as the most common arrhythmias encountered in primary cardiorespiratory arrest victims are ventricular fibrillation (VF) or pulseless ventricular tachycardia (pVT). Every minute of delay until defibrillation results in the number of successful cases returning to spontaneous circulation (ROSC) decreasing by approximately 10%.

Primary cardiorespiratory arrest is most common in adults but can occur in older children or children with congenital heart disease. Overall, however, the most common cause of cardiorespiratory arrest in children is secondary to other intercurrent illnesses.

Secondary cardiorespiratory arrest is usually due to hypoxia and reflects the limit of the body's ability to compensate for the effects of underlying illness or injury. Severe tissue hypoxia causes myocardial dysfunction, resulting in profound bradycardia, which typically deteriorates to asystole or pulseless electrical activity (PEA). Both PEA and asystole are associated with a poor outcome.

EPALS

Secondary cardiorespiratory arrest is rarely a sudden event, but follows a progressive deterioration. As respiratory and circulatory failure worsen (Figure 1.1), the body initially activates adaptive physiological responses compensating for the effects of the deterioration on vital organs (compensated respiratory or circulatory failure). These adaptive responses result in signs and symptoms that can be recognised, thereby providing an opportunity to intervene before further deterioration to cardiorespiratory arrest.

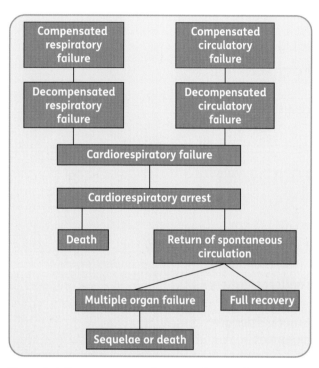

Figure 1.1 Consequences of progressive respiratory or circulatory failure

Outcome from secondary cardiorespiratory arrest

The outcome from secondary cardiorespiratory arrest is poor. Severe tissue hypoxia occurring before the heart stops means that all the vital organs are potentially seriously compromised; the heart finally arrests as a result of severe myocardial hypoxia.

Even if ROSC is achieved, morbidity and mortality remains high. Successful resuscitation from secondary cardiorespiratory arrest out-of-hospital is low (5–12% survival) and less than 5% of children will survive without neurological sequelae. In-hospital cardiac arrest (IHCA) results are better with a 70% ROSC rate but many children succumb to severe organ injury (e.g. brain, kidney) or multi-system organ failure 48–72 h post arrest; overall for IHCA 35–40% of children will survive to discharge. Resuscitation from respiratory arrest, when there is still cardiac output, is associated with much better (70–90%) good quality, long-term survival.

Anatomical and physiological considerations

The underlying anatomical and physiological differences between infants, young children and adults largely account for the difference in aetiology of cardiorespiratory arrest.

The key differences will be considered in order of management priority based on the ABCDE approach.

A	**Airway**
B	**Breathing**
C	**Circulation**
D	**Disability (mental status)**
E	**Exposure**

Airway

The infant/young child has an airway that is proportionately narrower and more susceptible to oedema and swelling than the adult. The absolute diameter of the airway is also smaller, and therefore respiratory infections account for a significantly higher level of morbidity and mortality in young children.

The effect of oedema and swelling can be seen in Poiseuille's law, which relates the resistance of the gas flowing through a tube (R) to its length (l), the viscosity of the gas (v) and the radius of the tube (r).

$$R = \frac{8l\,v}{\pi\, r^4}$$

Thus a small decrease in the airway radius (r) results in a huge increase (to the power of 4) of the resistance to flow of gases throughout the respiratory passages.

Relationship between head and neck

The infant's head is large in relation to the rest of their body. Since the occiput is protuberant, the head tends to flex on the neck when the infant is placed in a supine position. This leads to potential obstruction of the airway when the conscious level is reduced. With increasing age, the child's head becomes smaller in relation to their thorax, the neck lengthens and the larynx becomes more resistant to external pressure as tissues become less compliant.

Face and mouth

The infant's face is small and therefore the sizing of facemasks needs to be accurate otherwise it is difficult to achieve an effective seal. Additionally, pressure to the eyes can lead to damage and reflex bradycardia.

Inside the small mouth the tongue is relatively large. This combination means that airway obstruction is more likely in the unconscious infant/young child. The floor of the mouth is easily compressible; care is required to avoid compressing the soft tissues under the mandible to prevent airway obstruction when performing airway manoeuvres.

Nose and pharynx

The infant is a preferential nasal breather for the first six months or so of life. As a result, anything that causes nasal obstruction (e.g. anatomical abnormalities such as choanal atresia, copious secretions, nasogastric tubes or tapes) can lead to increased work of breathing and respiratory compromise.

The epiglottis in infants is larger and floppier than in adults. This means that it is vulnerable to damage by airway devices and manoeuvres.

The larynx

The larynx is higher in the infant compared to the older child and adult (where it is level with C5–6). Until about eight years, the child's larynx is funnel shaped, with its narrowest segment at the level of the cricoid cartilage, as opposed to the older child/adult, who has a larynx that is cylindrical in shape. The anatomical variations have the following practical implications:

- Blind finger sweeps to remove a foreign body must not be performed in young children with partial airway obstruction as these may convert a partial into a complete obstruction. The foreign body can become impacted into the narrowest part of the larynx (i.e. at the cricoid cartilage).

- The relatively large tongue may create airway obstruction as the epiglottis and larynx are higher in the neck.

- Control of the large tongue with a laryngoscope blade may be difficult.

- The high position of the larynx in an infant creates a sharp angle between the oropharynx and the glottis. Direct visualisation of the glottis with the laryngoscope is therefore difficult. It may be easier to use a straight blade rather than a curved blade to obtain a view, particularly in infants up to three months of age.

Breathing

Physiological considerations

The air-alveolar surface area for gas exchange in the lungs at birth is 3 m^2 compared with 70 m^2 in the adult. There is also a 10-fold increase in the number of small airways from birth to adulthood.

Normal respiratory function requires the movement of gas in and out of the lungs, and the exchange of oxygen (O_2) for carbon dioxide (CO_2) across the alveolar-capillary interface. Minute ventilation (the main determinant of CO_2 removal) depends upon the tidal volume (volume of gas with each breath) and the respiratory rate.

Minute ventilation = tidal volume x respiratory rate

Spontaneous tidal volume stays constant throughout life at 4–6 mL kg^{-1}. It can be qualitatively assessed by auscultation of the chest, listening to air entry in the upper and lower zones of both sides of the chest.

Infants and small children have a relatively small resting lung volume and hence a low oxygen reserve. In addition, they have a high rate of oxygen consumption. This combination results in rapid falls in blood oxygen levels when respiration is compromised.

Mechanics of breathing

As they age, the mechanics of children's breathing changes. The infant has ribs that are cartilaginous and pliable, while their intercostal muscles are weak and relatively ineffective. The main muscle of respiration is the diaphragm. During inspiration, the diaphragm descends towards the abdomen, generating a negative pressure, which draws air into the upper airway and the lungs. Mechanical impedance to the contraction of the diaphragm (e.g. gastric distension, intestinal obstruction) will result in ineffective ventilation, as will any obstruction of the airway (e.g. bronchiolitis, asthma or foreign body aspiration).

In older children, the more developed intercostal muscles contribute significantly to the mechanics of breathing. The ribs ossify and act as a secure anchor for the muscles, as well as forming a more rigid structure that is less likely to collapse in respiratory distress. In children above five years the presence of significant intercostal recession should therefore be considered as an ominous sign and indicative of serious respiratory compromise.

Respiratory rate

Normal respiration requires minimal effort and the resting respiratory rate varies with age. The infant has a relatively high metabolic rate, O_2 and CO_2 production, which is the main reason for their increased respiratory rates (Table 1.1). The respiratory rate also increases with agitation, anxiety and the presence of fever, therefore a record of respiratory rate as it changes over time is more useful than a single value.

Table 1.1 Respiratory rate ranges by age	
Age (years)	Respiratory rate (breaths min^{-1})
< 1	30–40
1–2	26–34
2–5	24–30
5–12	20–24
> 12	12–20

Circulation (and oxygen delivery)

The circulating volume of the newborn is 80 mL kg^{-1} and decreases with age to 60–70 mL kg^{-1} in adulthood. This means that the total circulating volume of an infant is very small (e.g. 240 mL in a newborn of 3 kg and 480 mL in a six month old with a weight of 6 kg). Relatively small losses can be a significantly high percentage of their total circulating volume; this is why apparently minor diarrhoeal illnesses can result in considerable morbidity and even mortality in infants and young children.

Oxygen delivery (DO$_2$) to cells in the body's tissues is determined by arterial oxygen content and cardiac output. Arterial O$_2$ content (CaO$_2$) is determined by circulating haemoglobin concentration and O$_2$ saturation and, to a small extent, the dissolved O$_2$ in the plasma.

Oxygen delivery to the body tissues

$$DO_2 = CaO_2 \times CO$$

DO$_2$ = oxygen delivery (mL min^{-1})
CaO$_2$ = arterial O$_2$ content (mL L^{-1})
CO   = cardiac output (L min^{-1})

Arterial oxygen content

$$CaO_2 = Hb \times 1.34 \times SaO_2$$

Hb = haemoglobin concentration (g L^{-1}).

The constant 1.34 is the O$_2$ carrying capacity of 1 g of haemoglobin (mL O$_2$ g Hb^{-1}).

Sa O$_2$ = oxygen saturation of haemoglobin (between 0 and 1 converted from percentage saturation value).

(SpO$_2$ is the peripheral oxygen saturation of blood which is, for practical purposes, almost identical to Sa O$_2$).

If either of the parameters of DO$_2$ (CaO$_2$ and CO) decreases and is not compensated for by an increase in the other parameter, tissue O$_2$ delivery decreases.

In respiratory failure, the fall in CaO$_2$ can be compensated by increasing CO.

A decrease in CO, as in circulatory failure, cannot be compensated by a rise in O$_2$ content. It is accompanied immediately by a decrease in tissue O$_2$ delivery. It is also important to compare DO$_2$ with O$_2$ demand, which may be higher than normal (as in septic shock).

Heart rate

Stroke volume (i.e. the amount of blood ejected with each contraction of the heart) is relatively small in infancy (1.5 mL kg^{-1} at birth) and increases along with heart size. However, the cardiac output relative to body weight is higher than at any other stage of life (300 mL kg^{-1} min^{-1}, decreasing to 100 mL kg^{-1} min^{-1} in adolescence and 70–80 mL kg^{-1} min^{-1} in adults).

Cardiac output is the product of stroke volume and heart rate, and so the high cardiac outputs in infants and young children are primarily achieved by rapid heart rates (Table 1.2).

Table 1.2 Heart rate ranges (beats min^{-1})			
Age	**Mean**	**Awake**	**Deep sleep**
Newborn – 3 months	140	85–205	80–140
3 months – 2 years	130	100–180	75–160
2–10 years	80	60–140	60–90
> 10 years	75	60–100	50–90

Since cardiac output is directly related to the heart rate, bradycardia is a serious event and should be treated vigorously. Systemic vascular resistance increases as the child ages and this is reflected in the changes seen in blood pressure (BP) ranges (Table 1.3).

Table 1.3 Blood pressure ranges by age systolic and mean				
Age	**Systolic BP 5th centile mmHg**	**Systolic BP 50th centile mmHg**	**Mean BP 5th centile mmHg**	**Mean BP 50th centile mmHg**
0–1 month	50	60	35	45
1–12 months	70	80	40	55
1–15 years	a) 1–10 yrs: 70 + 2 x age in yrs b) > 10 yrs: 90	90 + 2 x age in years	40 + 1.5 x age in years	55 + 1.5 x age in years
> 15 years	90	120	65	80

BP table revised 22 Dec 2016

In sick children and infants it is useful to consider the mean arterial blood pressure as an indicator of blood flow and it is believed to be a better indicator of tissue perfusion than systolic BP (as it accounts for the fact that two thirds of the cardiac cycle is spent in diastole). Mean arterial pressure (MAP) is derived from a patient's systolic blood pressure (SBP) and diastolic blood pressure (DBP). Since MAP is a product of cardiac output (CO) and systemic vascular resistance (SVR) (MAP = CO x SVR), variations in SVR make the relationship between MAP and CO often unreliable (e.g. a patient with a poor CO but high SVR such as a patient in cardiogenic shock may have an acceptable MAP but a CO that is too low to provide adequate perfusion to tissues). The MAP should be calculated in acute conditions by method below and compared to MAP expected (Table 1.3).

$$((2 \times diastolic) + systolic)) / 3 = MAP \ (mmHg)$$

Disability

The limited communication skills of infants and children have to be considered when attempting to assess neurological status. There is a tendency for ill children to regress to behaviour more befitting a younger child, especially if they are anxious or in pain. Effective pain control, empathy and appropriate language are therefore all essential factors when dealing with children. The presence of parents or other significant adults may help to alleviate many communication difficulties, as well as helping to allay fear and anxiety.

A rapid assessment of the child's conscious level can be obtained by determining the AVPU score (Chapter 2) or by the Glasgow Coma Scale score if doctors and nurses are familiar with its use; there is a modified scale for children under five years of age. Additionally, assessment of pupil size and reaction, and the child's posture, muscle tone and any focal signs should be noted to determine neurological status.

Exposure

To ensure that no significant clinical information is missed, examine the child fully by exposing their body. Appropriate measures to minimise heat loss (especially in infants) and respect dignity must be adopted at all times. The core body temperature should also be recorded and if necessary, appropriate measures to normalise it initiated.

Weight estimation

Medications are prescribed based on a child's body weight. In the emergency situation, it is often impractical to weigh the child, therefore an alternative method of estimating weight as accurately as possible is required. Examples are the Broselow tape or the Sandell tape, which relates the length of the child to their body weight, or centile charts that estimate weight against age.

An infant weights approximately 3 kg at birth and 10 kg at one year of age.

For the age group between one and ten years the following formula provides an approximation of weight:

$$\text{Weight (kg)} = (\text{Age in years} + 4) \times 2$$

The simplicity of this formula facilitates recollection under pressure and although the actual weight of obese children will be underestimated, drug dosage is usually based on lean body mass rather than actual mass. The action of intravenous resuscitation drugs in particular depends on plasma concentration so drug dosage based on lean body mass is appropriate.

Whatever method is used to establish the body weight of a child all healthcare professionals must be sufficiently familiar and competent in its use to be able to utilise it quickly and accurately. When using weight-based calculations don't administer a dose greater than the adult dose.

Causes of death and prevention

In the neonatal period, the most common aetiology of death is congenital anomaly, followed by adverse perinatal events and sudden infant death syndrome.

In infancy, congenital anomaly is still the leading cause of death, followed by respiratory and cardiovascular illness, infectious disease and trauma.

The most common cause of mortality in pre-school children (ages 1–4 years) is malignancy, followed by congenital anomalies, central nervous system disease, respiratory disease then trauma. For school-aged children between 5 and 9 years old malignancy is the major cause of death followed by central nervous system disease, respiratory disease, congenital anomalies then trauma. This is a change from 10 years ago when trauma was the leading cause of mortality in children over one year old. Trauma is the second highest cause of death in children from 10 to 14 years old. Accident prevention schemes need to be tailored to the different age groups. Such schemes depend on a combination of three elements:

- primary prevention – prevention of the accident (e.g. by using safe material in playgrounds, stair gates etc)

- secondary prevention – reducing the severity of an accident (e.g. by promoting the wearing of bicycle helmets)

- tertiary prevention – diminishing the consequence of the event by improving the effectiveness of emergency services after injury (e.g. taking part in a structured course such as EPALS).

Expected and unexpected death

The death of a child is emotionally distressing for parents, relatives and the healthcare professionals involved.

This latter group may include pre-hospital staff as well as those based at the hospital. An opportunity to hold a debriefing session for all staff after the death is important to allow them to air any concerns, feelings or emotions that arise from having delivered care to the child. Any member of the healthcare team should feel able to seek help and advice, from colleagues, their general practitioner (GP), bereavement counsellors or occupational health department if they feel they require it.

In any case of unexpected death, particularly when the cause is not clear, staff have a duty to make a referral to the coroner or procurator fiscal in Scotland and consider any safeguarding issues.

There are two interrelated processes for reviewing child deaths in the UK since April 2008: a rapid response by a group of key professionals who come together for the purpose of enquiring into and evaluating each unexpected death of a child and an overview of all child deaths (under 18 years) undertaken by child death overview panels (CDOPs), who report to the local safeguarding children's board (LSCB) of each area.

The GP, health visitor (for children under five years) and school nurse (for children over five years) must be informed about any paediatric deaths. In the UK, it is common practice to invite the parents approximately 4–6 weeks after the child's death to meet with the consultant in charge. This enables the parents to ask any questions and to receive information about the results of investigations that have taken place. The consultant would usually also be available to answer questions arising about the care that the child received (Chapter 13).

A child may have a condition for which it is agreed that resuscitation would not be beneficial. Looking after such a child and his family requires compassionate and considered management (palliative care) and is beyond the scope of the EPALS course.

In these circumstances advance care planning is advocated and the RC(UK) supports the use of the **ReSPECT** process and form: www.respectprocess.org.uk.

It is important to feel that the best possible care has been delivered as not all resuscitation attempts are successful. Early intervention based on the ABCDE approach will reduce the number of unexpected deaths. The EPALS course aims to provide this structured approach for the optimal care of children.

Summary learning

- **Children are more likely to suffer a secondary, rather than a primary cardiorespiratory arrest.**
- **Successful resuscitation from respiratory arrest, where there is still a cardiac output, is associated with 70–90% good quality, long-term survival.**
- **Survival from full secondary cardiorespiratory arrest without neurological sequelae is considerably less likely (< 5% out of hospital and approximately < 30% in hospital).**
- **The respiratory and circulatory anatomy and physiology of infants and young children influence both the aetiology and the management of their illnesses/injuries.**
- **The ABCDE approach is the basis of both the assessment and the management of seriously ill and/or injured children.**

My key take-home messages from this chapter

Further reading

Atkins DL, Everson-Stewart S, Sears GK, Daya M, Osmond MH, Warden CR, Berg RA; Resuscitation Outcomes Consortium Investigators. Epidemiology and outcomes from out-of-hospital cardiac arrest in children: the Resuscitation Outcomes Consortium Epistry-Cardiac Arrest. Circulation 2009; 24;119:1484-91.

Berg MD, Nadkarni VM, Berg RA. Cardioplumonary Resuscitation in Children. Curr Opin Crit Care. 2008;14:254-60.

Deasy C, Bernard SA, Cameron P et al. Epidemiology of paediatric out-of-hospital cardiac arrest in Melbourne, Resuscitation 2010; 81: 1095-1100.

Donoghue AJ, Nadkarni V, Berg RA, Osmond MH, Wells G, Nesbitt L, Stiell IG. Out-of-Hospital Pediatric Cardiac Arrest: An Epidemiologic Review and Assessment of Current Knowledge Ann Emerg Med. 2005;46:512-522.

Dudley NC, Hansen KW, Furnival RA, Donaldson AE, Van Wagenen KL, Scaife ER. The effect of family presence on the efficiency of pediatric trauma resuscitation. Ann Emerg Med 2009; 53: 777-784, e3.

Gupta P, Tang X, Gall CM, Lauer C, Rice TB, Wetzel RC. Epidemiology and outcomes of in-hopsital cardiac arrest in critically ill children across hospitals of varied center volume: A multi-center analysis. Resuscitation 2014;85:1473-9.

Kuisma M, Suominen P, Korpela R. Paesiatric out-of-hospital cardiac arrests: epidemiology and outcome. Resuscitation 1995;30:141-50.

Lopez-Herce J, Garcia C, Rodriguez-Nunez A, Dominguez P, Carillo A, Calvo C, Delgado MA. Long term outcome of paediatric cardiorespiratory arrest in Spain. Resuscitation 2005: 64:79-85.

Nadkarni VM, Larkin GL, Peberdy MA, Carey SM, Kaye W, Mancini ME, et al. First documented rhythm and clinical outcome from in-hospital cardiac arrest among children and adults. JAMA. 2006; 4;295:50-7.

Tibballs J, Kinney S. A prospective study of outcome of in-patient paediatric cardiopulmonary arrest. Resuscitation 2006;71;310-8.

Topjian AA, Nadkarni VM, Berg RA. Cardiopulmonary resuscitation in children. Curr Opin Crit Care. 2009; 15:203-8.

Safranek DJ, Eisenberg MS, Larsen MP. The epidemiology of cardiac arrest in young adults. Annals of emergency medicine 1992;21:1102-6.

Sirbaugh PE, Pepe PE, Shook JE, etal. A prospective, population based study of the demographics, epidemiology, management, and outcome of out-of-hospital pediatric cardiopulmonary arrest. Annals of emergency medicine 1999;33:174-84.

Go AS, Mozaffarian D, Roger VL et al (2014) Heart disease and stroke statistics-2014 update: a report from the American Heart Association. Circulation 129:e28-e292.

Naim MY, Burke RV, McNally BF et al. Association of Bystander Cardiopulmonary Resuscitation with Overall and Neurologically Favorable Survival after Pediatric Out-of-Hopsital Cardiac Arrest in the United States; a report from the Cardiac Arrest Registry to Enhance Survival Surveillance Registry (CARES). JAMA Pediatr 2017;17(2):133-141.,

Nitta M, Iwami T, Kitamura T, Nadkarni VM, Berg RA, Shimizu N, Ohta K, Nishiuchi T, Hayashi Y, Hiraide A, Tamai H, Kobayashi M, Morita H (2011) Age-specific differences in outcomes after out-of-hospital cardiac arrests. Pediatrics 128:e812-820.

Girotra S, Spertus JA, Li Y, Berg RA, Nadkarni VM, Chan PS; American Heart Association Get With the Guidelines–Resuscitation Investigators (2013) Survival trends in pediatric inhospital cardiac arrests: an analysis from Get With the Guidelines-Resuscitation. Circ Cardiovasc Qual Outcomes 6:42-49.

Haque IU, Zaritsky AL. Analysis for evidence for lower limit of systolic and mean arterial pressure in children, Paediatric critical care Medicine. 2007; 8, 2,138-122.

Website: The Children's Action Prevention Trust www.capt.org.uk

Website: Office for National Statistics. Child mortality statistics; Childhood, infant and perinatal 2013 (published March 2015) www.ons.gov.uk

Website: www.respectprocess.org.uk

Recognition and initial management of the seriously ill child

Contents

- Signs and symptoms of respiratory, circulatory and cardiorespiratory failure
- Parameters assessed during the ABCDE approach
- The ABCDE approach to the initial management of airway, breathing and circulation

Learning outcomes

To enable you to:

- Understand the importance of early recognition of the seriously ill child
- Describe the importance of the structured ABCDE approach to rapidly identify potential respiratory, circulatory and/or central neurological failure in the seriously ill child
- Consider the importance of the structured ABCDE approach to prioritise and assess effectiveness of initial management strategies

Early recognition of the seriously ill child

In children, cardiorespiratory arrest is usually due to hypoxia, reflecting the end of the body's ability to compensate for the effects of underlying illness or injury. The initial problem may originate from the airway, breathing or circulation. Irrespective of the primary aetiology, cardiorespiratory arrest in children is rarely a sudden event, but a progressive deterioration from combined respiratory and circulatory failure.

Early recognition and effective management of respiratory and/or circulatory failure will prevent the majority of paediatric cardiorespiratory arrests and thus reduce morbidity and mortality. It can also help identify children for whom attempted cardiorespiratory resuscitation may be inappropriate which can help facilitate suitable palliative care.

The principles outlined in this chapter apply to the seriously ill child in all environments (i.e. the acute hospital setting or out-of-hospital). Use of the structured ABCDE approach helps to ensure that potentially life-threatening problems are identified and managed in order of their priority.

A: Airway problems

A review of practical airway management procedures is provided in Chapter 4.

Causes of upper airway obstruction

Airway obstruction can be partial or complete, sudden or insidious, progressive or recurrent. Respiratory rate and work of breathing generally increase in airway obstruction. When assessing airway patency, **chest movement does not guarantee that the airway is clear.** Air entry needs to be assessed as well by looking, listening and feeling for air movement, and by chest auscultation.

Initially, airway obstruction is often partial but can lead to respiratory failure, exhaustion, secondary apnoea and eventually hypoxic brain damage. Additionally, partial airway obstruction can rapidly become total, and result in cardiorespiratory arrest.

Congenital abnormalities such as choanal atresia or Pierre-Robin syndrome can be initially managed by use of an appropriate airway adjunct to open the airway and buy time, prior to definitive treatment.

Depression of the central nervous system can cause loss of airway control as protective upper airway reflexes and muscle tone are lost. This may be compounded in the infant due to the age related anatomical features. The pronounced occiput and short neck causes head flexion in the supine position and, together with the proportionately large tongue, can quickly lead to airway obstruction in the unconscious infant.

Causes of central nervous system depression include hypoxia following decompensated respiratory or circulatory failure, head trauma, metabolic disorders (e.g. hypoglycaemia, inborn errors of metabolism), hypercapnia, alcohol and medications (e.g. opiates, benzodiazepines). Airway obstruction due to these causes may not be accompanied by tachypnoea or increased work of breathing.

Table 2.1 Causes of airway obstruction

- Congenital abnormality (e.g. choanal atresia, Pierre-Robin syndrome)
- Secretions (e.g. vomit, blood)
- Respiratory tract infections (swelling or mucus secretions)
- Pharyngeal swelling (e.g. oedema, infection)
- Epiglottitis
- Laryngotracheobronchitis (croup)
- Nasal feeding tubes
- Oxygen delivery devices (e.g. nasal cannulae)
- Foreign body (e.g. food, toy, orthodontic appliances)
- Central nervous system depression (loss of muscle tone)
- Trauma (facial or throat)

Recognition of upper airway obstruction

Airway obstruction may be demonstrated by difficulty in breathing and/or increased respiratory effort. In a conscious child there may be visible distress. There may be additional respiratory noises, such as inspiratory stridor, if the obstruction is partial. Causes are seen in Table 2.1.

Management of upper airway obstruction

The treatment of partial airway obstruction is to maintain airway patency and ensure that it does not become totally occluded. This may be achieved by head positioning,

clearance of any secretions or foreign bodies, and summoning further assistance as indicated.

In patients with airway obstruction, delivery of supplemental oxygen is advised as early as possible, to minimise the potential effects of hypoxia.

The conscious child will usually adopt a position that optimises airway patency. If the child is stable, and deterioration is considered unlikely, he should be left with his parents/carers who can help administer oxygen and minimise stress and anxiety. Feeding should be avoided, and any fever treated to reduce increased metabolic demand. If there is a decreased level of consciousness, airway compromise must be assumed. The management priorities are to get more help whilst safeguarding the airway and preventing complications such as aspiration of gastric contents, by placing the child in the recovery position or supporting the head-up position.

Basic airway opening manoeuvres (e.g. head tilt and chin lift or jaw thrust) should be used. Adjuncts such as oro/nasopharyngeal airways can also be used until more experienced help is available. Advanced emergency airway management may involve insertion of a tracheal tube, laryngeal mask airway (LMA) or cricothyroidotomy, although the latter will only provide temporary oxygenation until a definitive airway can be achieved.

B: Breathing problems

In all seriously ill or injured children, the priority is for the appropriate management of the airway and ventilation (breathing).

Causes of breathing (respiratory) problems

Respiratory failure can result from acute or chronic breathing inadequacy. Movement of air into and out of the lungs (ventilation) and/or gas exchange at the alveolar capillary interface is compromised. The underlying problem may be due to lung pathology (i.e. congenital or acquired diseases or trauma) or have a non-respiratory origin (e.g. circulatory failure, metabolic disorder, neurological problem).

Failure of ventilation results in CO_2 accumulation and reduced oxygen levels. Reduced gas exchange across the alveolar-capillary interface is often a result of fluid accumulation within the alveoli (pulmonary oedema or infection) and results in a fall in arterial O_2 levels and increased lung stiffness (i.e. decreased lung compliance). Other common causes of the failure of gas exchange include bronchospasm and atelectasis, which are also associated with stiff lungs. The arterial O_2 levels fall, which stimulate breathing via peripheral chemoreceptors (the aortic and carotid bodies).

Arterial CO_2 levels may initially be normal or even low due to an increased respiratory rate, although they will rise stimulating the respiratory centre to increase the respiratory rate further as failure worsens. The work of breathing then increases not only due to the increased respiratory rate but also due to the increased lung stiffness.

Increased arterial CO_2 levels may also result in tachycardia, vasodilatation and bounding pulses, but these are unreliable findings.

The respiratory rate can be classified as abnormal if it is too rapid (tachypnoea), too slow (bradypnoea) or absent (apnoea). Respiratory distress is a clinical syndrome, which reflects increased work of breathing, often associated with attempts to increase tidal volume and can be associated with either tachypnoea or bradypnoea.

As the work of breathing increases, an increased proportion of the cardiac output is diverted to the respiratory muscles with a consequent increase in the amount of CO_2 produced.

Ultimately, if decompensation occurs, the respiratory system is unable to provide sufficient oxygen for tissue requirements, anaerobic metabolism occurs and respiratory acidosis is complicated by metabolic acidosis.

Recognition of respiratory failure

From a physiological viewpoint, respiratory failure is usually defined as failure of the respiratory system to maintain an arterial oxygen level (PaO_2) > 9 kPa with 21% inspired O_2 (air) and/or arterial carbon dioxide level of ($PaCO_2$) < 6.5 kPa. This definition requires arterial blood gas analysis. However, a PaO_2 of 9 kPa corresponds approximately to a peripheral oxygen saturation (SpO_2) of approximately 90%.

A child with respiratory distress may be able to maintain their arterial blood gas values within relatively normal limits by increasing their respiratory effort. It is therefore important to evaluate whether the child's situation is stable or if decompensation to respiratory failure is imminent. This evaluation requires knowledge of the signs and symptoms of respiratory distress and/or respiratory failure. When the compensatory mechanisms fail, deterioration is rapid and imminent cardiorespiratory arrest must be anticipated.

Warning signs are:

- decreased level of consciousness
- hypotonia
- decreased respiratory effort
- cyanosis or extreme pallor (despite oxygen being given)
- sweating
- bradycardia.

In children, recognition of respiratory failure is based on the full assessment of respiratory effort and efficacy, and the identification of evidence of respiratory inadequacy on major organs.

Work of breathing

Evidence of increased work of breathing is based on observation of the following:

- increased respiratory rate
- intercostal recession
- sternal recession
- subcostal recession
- use of accessory muscles (e.g. nasal flaring)
- head bobbing.

Respiratory rate

Tachypnoea is frequently the first indication of respiratory insufficiency. Normal respiratory rates vary with age and this must be considered when determining the presence of tachypnoea (Table 2.2).

| Table 2.2 Respiratory rate ranges by age ||
Age (years)	Respiratory rate (breaths min⁻¹)
< 1	30–40
1–2	26–34
2–5	24–30
5–12	20–24
> 12	12–20

Changes in respiratory rate over time are very important. An increasing respiratory rate represents increasing physiological compensation to offset the deterioration in respiratory function. A sudden reduction in the respiratory rate in an acutely ill child is an ominous sign and may be a pre-terminal event. Causes may include exhaustion, central nervous system depression or hypothermia. Fatigue is always an important consideration in children: an infant with a respiratory rate of 80 min⁻¹ will tire quickly.

Recession

Recession (or retractions) may be sternal, subcostal or intercostal. The degree of recession gives an indication of the severity of respiratory disorder. Infants and young children can exhibit significant recession with relatively mild to moderate respiratory compromise, owing to their highly compliant chest wall. However, in children over approximately five years (by which age the chest wall is less compliant) recession is a sign of significant respiratory compromise.

Use of accessory muscles

When the work of breathing is increased, the sternocleidomastoid muscles in the neck are often used as accessory respiratory muscles. In infants, this may cause the head to bob up and down with each breath. This 'head bobbing' actually reduces the efficiency of each breath.

'See-saw' respiration

A breathing pattern, described as 'see-saw' respiration, is sometimes observed in severe respiratory compromise. It is the paradoxical movement of the abdomen during inspiration (i.e. the abdomen expands and the thorax retracts as the diaphragm contracts). This is inefficient respiration because the tidal volume is reduced, despite the increased muscular effort.

Inspiratory and expiratory noises

Normally, the airway above the thoracic inlet (extrathoracic) narrows and the airway below (intrathoracic) widens during the inspiratory phase of breathing. This pattern reverses on expiration. Observing the timing of an abnormal noise can indicate the site of airway obstruction. The presence of a high-pitched inspiratory noise (stridor) is characteristic of an upper airway (extrathoracic) obstruction and is due to rapid, turbulent flow through a narrowed portion of the upper tracheal airway. In severe obstruction, the stridor may also occur on expiration (biphasic stridor) but is usually less pronounced than it is during inspiration.

Wheezing is generally an expiratory noise. It is indicative of lower (intrathoracic) airway narrowing, usually at bronchiolar level, and may be audible with the ear, or only on chest auscultation with a stethoscope.

The volume of airway noises is not indicative of the severity of respiratory compromise; diminishing noises may be indicative of increasing airway obstruction or exhaustion of the child.

Grunting

Grunting is mainly heard in neonates and small infants, but can also occur in young children. It is the result of exhaling against a partially closed glottis, and is an attempt to generate a positive end-expiratory pressure thus preventing airway collapse at the end of expiration. Grunting is generally associated with 'stiff' lungs (e.g. respiratory distress syndrome, pulmonary oedema, atelectasis). Regardless of the underlying condition, grunting is an indication of severe respiratory compromise.

Nostril flaring

Flaring of the nostrils is often seen in infants and young children with increased respiratory effort.

Position

Children in respiratory distress will usually adopt a position to maximise their respiratory capacity. In upper airway obstruction, they often adopt a 'sniffing the morning air' position to optimise their upper airway patency. In generalised or lower respiratory problems, children often sit forward, supporting their weight on their arms, and holding on to (or wrapping their arms around) their knees. This position results in a degree of shoulder girdle 'splinting', which enhances accessory muscle use. The child should be supported in the position of optimal airway

maximisation/comfort for them and have oxygen therapy given accordingly.

The degree of respiratory distress generally provides clinical evidence of the severity of respiratory insufficiency. However, there are three general exceptions to this (Table 2.3).

Table 2.3 Exceptions to increased work of breathing in respiratory failure

1. Exhaustion – children who have had severe respiratory compromise for some time may have progressed to decompensation and no longer show signs of increased work of breathing

   Exhaustion is a pre-terminal event

2. Neuromuscular diseases (e.g. muscular dystrophy)

3. Central respiratory depression – reduced respiratory drive results in respiratory inadequacy (e.g. encephalopathy, medications such as morphine)

Efficacy of breathing

The infant's relatively higher metabolic rate and oxygen consumption accounts for their increased respiratory rates (Table 2.2). Thus the effectiveness of breathing can be assessed by respiratory rate together with tidal volume, which in turn is evaluated by observation of chest movement, palpation, auscultation and percussion. Additional information can be easily obtained by non-invasive pulse oximetry.

Chest movement, palpation and percussion

Observation of chest movement demonstrates the extent and symmetry of chest expansion. As well as revealing increased work of breathing, observing the movement of the chest wall can help identify diminished or asymmetrical respiratory effort.

Palpation of the chest wall may identify deformities, surgical emphysema or crepitus.

Percussion of the chest wall can demonstrate areas of collapse (dullness) or hyper-resonance (e.g. in pneumothorax).

Chest auscultation

When listening with a stethoscope, air entry should be heard in all areas of the lungs. Volume of air movement occurring with inspiration and expiration can be estimated by auscultation. It is useful to compare the areas on one side of the chest with the other.

A very quiet or near silent chest indicates a dangerously reduced tidal volume and is an ominous sign.

Pulse oximetry

A pulse oximeter should be used on any child with potential respiratory failure to provide an assessment of the patient's arterial oxygen saturation.

Without pulse oximetry it is not always clinically possible to detect that the child has a decreased arterial oxygen saturation of haemoglobin (SaO_2) until the saturation is between 80–85%. Pulse oximetry is simple to use, relatively cheap, non-invasive and provides an immediate, objective measure of arterial blood oxygen saturation. An arterial oxygen saturation (SpO_2) of < 90% in air or the inability to raise SpO_2 > 94% with supplemental oxygen indicates respiratory failure. Below 70% the displayed values are highly unreliable.

Most pulse oximeters have an audible tone related to the SpO_2, with a decreasing tone reflecting increasing hypoxaemia. The pulse rate is also usually displayed. A poor signal indicates a low blood pressure or poor tissue perfusion.

Pulse oximeter readings must not be used in isolation: it is vital to interpret them in light of the clinical picture and alongside other investigations, and potential sources of error. Pulse oximetry provides only a measure of oxygen saturation, not content, and thus gives no indication of actual tissue oxygenation. Furthermore, it provides no information on adequacy of ventilation. A patient may be breathing inadequately and have a high carbon dioxide level despite a normal oxygen saturation. Arterial blood gases are needed in critically ill patients to assess oxygenation and ventilation.

Pulse oximetry has four main uses:

1. Detection of/screening for hypoxaemia

2. Targeting oxygen therapy

3. Routine monitoring during anaesthesia

4. Diagnostic (e.g. sleep apnoea).

There are several acknowledged sources of error with pulse oximetry:

- presence of other haemoglobins: carboxyhaemoglobin (carbon monoxide poisoning) and methaemoglobin (congenital or acquired)

- surgical and imaging dyes: methylene blue, indocyanine green and indigo carmine cause falsely low saturation readings

- nail varnish (especially blue, black and green)

- high-ambient light levels (fluorescent and xenon lamps)

- motion artefact.

Reduced pulse volume:

- hypotension

- low cardiac output

- vasoconstriction

- hypothermia.

Pulse oximeters are not affected by:

- anaemia (reduced haemoglobin concentration)

- jaundice (hyperbilirubinaemia)

- skin pigmentation.

Pulse oximetry does not provide a reliable signal during CPR.

Central Cyanosis

Central cyanosis appears when the SpO_2 is < 80% (it indicates that desaturated haemoglobin is > 5 g dL^{-1}). The absence of cyanosis, particularly in anaemic patients, does not imply that the blood oxygen levels are normal. Cyanosis is an inconsistent sign of respiratory failure. It is most apparent on the mucosae of the mouth and in the nail beds. Cyanosis limited to the extremities is usually due to circulatory failure (peripheral cyanosis) rather than to respiratory failure (central cyanosis). Hypoxia may also cause vasoconstriction and skin pallor, which will mask cyanosis. However, in a child with acute respiratory compromise, the development of central cyanosis is a late indication of severe hypoxia and is a pre-terminal sign.

Effects of respiratory inadequacy on other body organs

Ongoing respiratory compromise rapidly affects other body organs/systems.

Heart rate

Hypoxia initially causes tachycardia. As this is a non-specific sign it needs to be considered alongside other clinical signs. Severe or prolonged hypoxia ultimately leads to bradycardia and therefore it is important to observe for trends rather than absolute values in heart rate. In a severely hypoxic child, bradycardia is a pre-terminal sign.

Skin perfusion

Hypoxia produces vasoconstriction and pallor of the skin. As their clinical condition deteriorates, the child's colour may become mottled before cyanosis appears centrally (lips and mouth).

Conscious level

Hypoxia and/or hypercapnia initially lead to agitation and/or drowsiness. Ongoing cerebral hypoxia ultimately results in loss of consciousness. In infants and young children, initial cerebral hypoxia may be difficult to detect but their parents/carers frequently report that the baby/child is not responding to them as usual. This information is important and should not be ignored. The level of consciousness should be assessed using the AVPU score (Table 2.4).

Generalised hypotonia also accompanies cerebral hypoxia.

Table 2.4 The level of consciousness

A	**ALERT**
V	**responds to VOICE**
P	**responds to PAIN**
U	**UNRESPONSIVE to painful stimuli**

The management of respiratory compromise

The treatment of breathing problems is dependent on achieving a patent airway and effective delivery of oxygen. The method of oxygen administration will vary according to the child's clinical condition and age. Children who have adequate spontaneous breathing should have high-flow oxygen delivered in a manner that is non-threatening (when agitated the child's airflow will become turbulent and resistance to flow will increase) and best tolerated by them (e.g. from a free-flow device held by their parents, a non-rebreathing facemask or nasal cannulae).

When breathing is inadequate (or absent) high-flow oxygen should be delivered by ventilation with a bag and mask system. In situations where the child is exhausted and is likely to need ongoing respiratory support, tracheal intubation may be indicated.

Targeted oxygen therapy

In critically ill patients, those presenting with acute hypoxaemia or in the peri-arrest situation, give high-concentration oxygen immediately. Give this initially with an oxygen mask and reservoir ('non-rebreathing' mask) and an oxygen flow of 12–15 L min^{-1}. During cardiorespiratory arrest use 100% oxygen to maximise arterial oxygen content and delivery to the tissues.

When the oxygen saturation of arterial blood can be monitored reliably, adjust the inspired oxygen concentration to maintain a SpO_2 of 94–98%. If pulse oximetry (with a reliable reading) is unavailable, continue oxygen via a reservoir mask until definitive monitoring or assessment of oxygenation is available. All critically ill patients will need arterial blood gas sampling and analysis as soon as possible. Evidence suggests hypoxaemia and, particularly in newborns, hyperoxaemia (PaO_2 > 20 kPa) in the post-resuscitation phase may lead to worse outcomes than those in whom normoxaemia is maintained.

C: Circulatory problems

The appropriate management of the airway and ventilation (breathing) is the priority in all seriously ill children and should be addressed before considering their circulatory status.

Circulatory failure and shock

Shock is a clinical state where the delivery of oxygenated blood and associated delivery of nutrients (e.g. glucose) to the body tissues is inadequate for metabolic demand. Additionally, the removal of cellular waste (e.g. CO_2, lactic acid) may also be impaired. Circulatory failure refers to insufficient blood being delivered to the body's tissues.

Shock may occur with increased, normal or decreased cardiac output (CO) or blood pressure (BP). Initially, the child's body can physiologically compensate for reduced tissue perfusion. However, when blood pressure starts to fall, as seen in circulatory failure, perfusion of the vital organs (e.g. brain, myocardium, kidneys) becomes increasingly compromised. Inadequate tissue blood flow results in anaerobic metabolism and lactic acid accumulation occurs. The resultant cell damage may be irreversible. It is therefore very important to promptly recognise and treat any child with compensated circulatory failure, to prevent deterioration to a decompensated state.

Compensated circulatory failure may have a normal blood pressure, but signs of abnormal perfusion, tachycardia, poor skin perfusion (prolonged capillary refill time), weak peripheral pulse, tachypnoea and reduced urine output are observed.

Decompensated circulatory failure is present when hypotension develops and vital organ perfusion is compromised. The clinical signs of inadequate tissue perfusion are much more apparent.

Aetiology of shock

Shock can arise from circulatory or respiratory failure. Most children with sustained shock, whatever its aetiology, have some degree of cardiovascular dysfunction requiring more than one type of treatment (i.e. managing the airway, breathing and circulation).

Although CO is usually decreased in circulatory failure, in septic and anaphylactic shock CO may be increased. In this case the systemic vascular resistance (SVR) is low and although the child appears to be well perfused (so called warm shock) with bounding peripheral pulses and an increased pulse pressure (the difference between the systolic and diastolic BP), the metabolic requirements of the tissues are not being met due to a mismatch between blood flow and metabolic demand.

The most common causes of circulatory failure in children are hypovolaemia, sepsis or anaphylaxis.

Hypovolaemic shock: Characterised by decreased circulating volume (preload). It may result from severe fluid loss (as in dehydration) or haemorrhage.

Distributive shock: Typified by inadequate distribution of blood, so that the blood flow is insufficient for the metabolic demand of the tissues (e.g. anaphylaxis, sepsis or neurogenic).

Cardiogenic shock: Circulatory failure is less commonly the result of a primary cardiac problem due to congenital or acquired heart disease (e.g. cardiomyopathy, myocarditis or following cardiac surgery).

Obstructive shock: An uncommon cause of circulatory failure due to obstruction of blood flow to/from the heart (e.g. tension pneumothorax, cardiac tamponade or constrictive pericarditis).

Dissociative shock: Characterised by insufficient oxygen carrying capacity of the blood (e.g. anaemia or carbon monoxide poisoning).

Evaluation of the circulatory system

Oxygen delivery to the tissues is dependent on the arterial oxygen content and the CO. The CO is the product of the blood volume ejected from the left ventricle with each contraction and the heart rate.

> ### Cardiac output
> **CO = HR x SV**
>
> CO = cardiac output.
>
> HR = heart rate.
>
> SV (stroke volume) = blood volume ejected with each contraction.

> ### Blood pressure
> **BP = CO x SVR**
>
> BP = blood pressure.
>
> SVR = systemic vascular resistance.

Of the variables affecting or affected by CO (Figure 2.1), some can be easily measured (HR and BP) and others (SV and SVR) must be indirectly assessed by examining the amplitude and quality of pulses, and the adequacy of end-organ perfusion (mental status, capillary refill time, skin temperature and, when available, urine output).

A low SVR or CO should be suspected if the systolic BP is below the normal range for the child's age.

Recognition of circulatory failure

In children, the recognition of circulatory failure is based on a complete cardiovascular assessment, looking for the effects of any circulatory insufficiency on major organs.

Parameters evaluated include:

- heart rate
- pulse volume
- capillary refill time
- blood pressure

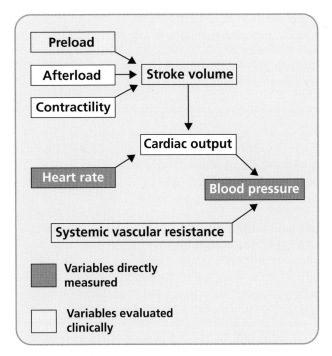

Figure 2.1 Evaluation of cardiovascular relationships

- filling pressure (liver size in infants or jugular vein filling in older children)

- end organ perfusion status.

Heart rate

The heart rate initially rises to maintain cardiac output.

Sinus tachycardia is a common response to many situations (e.g. pain, anxiety, fever) but it is also seen in hypoxia, hypercapnia and hypovolaemia. When tachycardia is accompanied by other signs of circulatory insufficiency, it is evidence of the body's attempts at physiological compensation. Neonates have limited cardiac reserve; they increase their CO primarily by increasing heart rate rather than stroke volume (SV). They develop tachycardia as the first response to hypoxia.

When the increased heart rate is unable to maintain adequate tissue perfusion, the tissue hypoxia and acidosis result in bradycardia. The presence of bradycardia is a pre-terminal sign, indicating that cardiorespiratory arrest is imminent.

Pulse volume

Feeling for the volume (or amplitude) of central pulses (e.g. femoral, carotid, brachial) gives a subjective indication of SV; as SV decreases, so does the pulse amplitude. In progressive circulatory failure, the pulse amplitude diminishes, becomes weak and thready before finally, it is impalpable. Simultaneous palpation and comparison of central and peripheral pulses (e.g. radial and carotid) may be useful. Peripheral pulses decrease in amplitude earlier than central ones. Note that caution is required in their interpretation when vasoconstriction is present (e.g. ambient temperature is low, or in an anxious or pyrexial child).

The presence or absence of peripheral pulses is neither a specific nor sensitive indicator of circulatory compromise, but is useful in conjunction with other clinical signs. However, diminishing central pulses are a pre-terminal sign, indicating that cardiorespiratory arrest is imminent.

Capillary refill and skin colour

The skin of a healthy child is warm to touch unless the ambient temperature is low. Their capillary refill time (CRT) is normally < 2 s, but when there is decreased skin perfusion, the CRT is prolonged.

Evaluation of CRT is best performed by applying cutaneous pressure on the centre of the sternum for 5 s. Following removal of the pressure, the blanching of the skin should disappear within 2 s. A slower refill time (i.e. prolonged CRT) is indicative of poor skin perfusion. A pyrexial child with hypovolaemia will have a prolonged CRT, despite having a raised body temperature. A low ambient temperature or poor local lighting conditions reduces the accuracy of CRT. The CRT should be considered in context of the accompanying cardiovascular signs.

Initially, hypoxia produces vasoconstriction and hence the child appears pale. As their clinical condition deteriorates, the child's colour becomes mottled and ultimately cyanosed. Cyanosis due to circulatory failure is initially peripheral, whereas hypoxaemia due to respiratory failure results in central cyanosis.

Peripheral vasoconstriction and decreased perfusion may also be indicated by a demarcation line between warm and cold skin. This can be detected by running the back of your hand up the child's limb. The demarcation line will travel towards the trunk over time if the child's condition is deteriorating, and vice versa if it is improving.

Blood pressure

In most forms of shock, the BP is initially maintained within the normal range (Table 2.5) for the child as a result of the body's compensatory mechanisms (e.g. tachycardia, vasoconstriction, increased myocardial contractility). Only when compensation is no longer possible, does hypotension occur and a decompensated state results.

In hypovolaemia, approximately 40% of the child's total circulating volume can be lost before hypotension occurs.

This means that BP only drops at a late stage in hypovolaemia (e.g. trauma, diarrhoeal illness, gut necrosis). It is therefore important that compensated circulatory failure is detected and managed at an early stage (i.e. before BP drops and decompensation occurs).

In children over one year, BP limits can be estimated by the formulae in Table 2.5.

In full term neonates, the lower limit for systolic BP is 50 mmHg and for infants, from 1–12 months, it is 70 mmHg.

Regardless of the method used to obtain the BP (auscultatory or oscillometric) it is important that the appropriate cuff size is used. The cuff width should be > 80% of the child's upper arm length, and the bladder cover more than 40% of the circumference of their arm. The same size cuff should be used on each occasion that the BP is measured.

Hypotension is a sign of physiological decompensation and indicates imminent cardiorespiratory arrest.

Filling pressure

If the heart is unable to effectively pump the blood returned to it, either because there is fluid overload or because the heart is failing, the pressure in the veins supplying the heart is raised. This is manifested by crackles at the lung bases, distention of the jugular veins in older children or enlargement of the liver in infants. Observation of these signs forms part of the reassessment following a fluid bolus.

Effects of circulatory inadequacy on other body organs

Ongoing circulatory compromise rapidly affects other body organs/systems:

Respiratory system

The metabolic acidosis that results from circulatory compromise leads to tachypnoea. However, there will not initially be other signs of increased work of breathing.

Conscious level

Hypoxia and/or hypercapnia initially lead to agitation and/or drowsiness. Progressive cerebral hypoxia ultimately results in loss of consciousness.

Age	Systolic BP 5th centile mmHg	Systolic BP 50th centile mmHg	Mean BP 5th centile mmHg	Mean BP 50th centile mmHg
0–1 month	50	60	35	45
1–12 months	70	80	40	55
1–15 years	a) 1–10 yrs: 70 + 2 x age in yrs b) > 10 yrs: 90	90 + 2 x age in years	40 + 1.5 x age in years	55 + 1.5 x age in years
> 15 years	90	120	65	80

Table 2.5 Blood pressure ranges by age systolic and mean

BP table revised 22 Dec 2016

In infants and young children, initial cerebral hypoxia may be difficult to detect but their parents/carers frequently report that the baby/child is not responding to them as usual and, as in respiratory failure, this information should not be ignored. The level of consciousness should be assessed by the AVPU score.

Generalised hypotonia also accompanies cerebral hypoxia.

Urine output

Information regarding the degree of reduced renal perfusion can be obtained by measuring the output of urine. A urinary output of < 2 mL kg^{-1} h^{-1} in infants or < 1 mL kg^{-1} h^{-1} in children older than one year, is an indication of inadequate renal perfusion. Asking parents/carers about the child's urine output (e.g. the number of wet nappies; normal would be at least six wet nappies per day) may reveal a history of oliguria or anuria.

Management of circulatory compromise

The treatment of circulatory problems is dependent on achieving a patent airway and effectively managing ventilation with appropriate delivery of high-flow oxygen before turning attention to circulatory procedures.

Immediately life-threatening causes of circulatory failure (e.g. massive or continuing haemorrhage, tension pneumothorax) must be sought and urgently treated.

Insertion of at least one large bore vascular cannula should be performed rapidly. This can be achieved by either intravenous or intraosseous routes.

Unless contraindicated (e.g. cardiac failure) volume replacement should be started using 20 mL kg^{-1} boluses of isotonic salt solution (i.e. 0.9% saline). Glucose containing fluids with low sodium levels should NEVER be used for resuscitation, only to correct for low blood glucose levels.

The use of vasoactive medications may be needed (circulatory access procedures, fluids and medications are in Chapter 5).

Cardiorespiratory failure

Signs of cardiorespiratory failure include alteration of consciousness, hypotonia, tachycardia, decreased central pulses and absent peripheral pulses. Bradycardia, hypotension, bradypnoea, gasping and apnoea are terminal events preceding imminent cardiorespiratory arrest.

If any of the following signs are present, immediate intervention should be undertaken:

- coma or alteration of consciousness

- exhaustion

- cyanosis

- tachypnoea (RR > 60 min^{-1})

- HR < 100 min^{-1} for newborn

- HR > 180 min^{-1} or < 80 min^{-1} before one year (note: chest compressions in all ages should be started if HR < 60 min^{-1})

- HR > 160 min^{-1} or < 60 min^{-1} after one year

- seizures.

A rapid assessment must be made of every child in whom respiratory, circulatory or cardiorespiratory failure is suspected.

D: Disability – central neurological assessment

Following the appropriate management of the child's airway, ventilation and circulation, their neurological status should be evaluated.

Whilst both respiratory and circulatory failure can have central neurological effects, some neurological conditions may affect the respiratory and circulatory systems (Table 2.6).

Table 2.6 Causes of altered conscious level

- Respiratory failure
- Circulatory failure
- Neurological disorders (e.g status epilepticus, meningitis, encephalitis)
- Hypoglycaemia
- Head injury
- Raised intracranial pressure
- Drugs (e.g. opiates, alcohol)
- Metabolic disorders

Neurological function

Conscious level

A rapid assessment of the child's conscious level can be determined by the AVPU score.

If required, a painful stimulus should be delivered either by applying pressure to the supraorbital ridge or rubbing the sternum. A child who is responsive to painful (P) stimuli has a significant degree of neurological derangement equivalent to a Glasgow Coma Scale score of approximately 8.

Pupils

The size and reactivity of pupils can be affected by a number of things, including medications, intracranial pressure and cerebral lesions. Important signs to look for are dilatation, inequality and non-reactivity of the child's pupils. These features potentially indicate serious brain dysfunction.

Posture

Seriously ill children become hypotonic and floppy. However, if there is serious brain dysfunction, stiff posturing may be demonstrated. This posturing (which may only be evident when a painful stimulus is applied) can be decorticate (flexed arms and extended legs) or decerebrate (extended arms and legs); both indicate serious brain dysfunction and may be signs of raised intracranial pressure.

Blood glucose

Bed-side blood sugar estimation should be performed in all seriously ill children. The increased metabolic rate associated with acute illness leads to increased use of glucose. Infants and small children do not have large glycogen liver stores which can be broken down to generate more glucose and therefore may become hypoglycaemic with any acute illness particularly when oral intake is reduced.

Effects on other systems of central neurological failure

Central neurological dysfunction may affect other body systems.

Respiratory system

Comatose children with brain dysfunction may exhibit abnormal respiratory patterns (e.g. hyperventilation, Cheyne-Stoke respiratory pattern (alternate periods of hyperventilation and apnoea) or complete apnoea).

Circulatory system

Raised intracranial pressure causes the Cushing's triad (i.e. abnormal breathing pattern with bradycardia and hypertension). This is a late and pre-terminal sign of neurological failure.

Management of neurological compromise

The initial steps in management of any child with a reduced conscious level must always be to maintain an open airway, ensure adequate ventilation and oxygenation, and support circulation in order to maintain cerebral oxygenation and perfusion.

Other causes of neurological compromise must then be considered and specific investigations and treatments given as indicated (e.g. glucose for hypoglycaemia, CT scanning if head injury or cerebral infections are suspected).

E: Exposure

To ensure that no additional significant clinical information (e.g. rashes) is missed, examine the child fully by exposing their body. Appropriate measures to minimise heat loss (especially in infants) and respect dignity must be adopted at all times.

The ABCDE approach

In all seriously ill or injured children, the underlying principles of assessment, initial management and ongoing reassessments are the same. They are based on the systematic ABCDE approach.

A	**Airway**
B	**Breathing**
C	**Circulation**
D	**Disability (mental status)**
E	**Exposure**

General principles of the ABCDE approach

- Ensure personal safety.

- Observe the child generally to determine the overall level of illness (i.e. do they look seriously unwell; are they interacting with parents/care providers).

- Speak to the child and assess the appropriateness of their response; ask the parents about the child's 'usual' behaviour.

- If they are unconscious and unresponsive to your voice, administer tactile stimulation. If they respond by speaking or crying, this indicates that they have a patent airway, are breathing and have cerebral perfusion. Regardless of the child's response to initial stimulation, you should move on to full assessment of ABCDE.

- Appropriate high-flow oxygen delivery should be commenced immediately.

- Vital sign monitoring should be requested early (ECG, SpO_2 and non-invasive BP monitoring).

- Circulatory access should be achieved as soon as possible. Blood test investigations and a bedside glucose estimation should be obtained.

Summary learning

- **Early recognition of the seriously ill child prevents the majority of cardiorespiratory arrests, thus reducing morbidity and mortality.**

- **The structured ABCDE approach helps ensure that potentially life-threatening problems are identified and dealt with in order of priority.**

Table 2.7 Specific assessments and actions in initial ABCDE approach

Assessment	Information sought	Possible resultant actions
On approaching the child	**Note:** • **General appearance** • **Interaction with parent/caregiver**	
A Airway patency	Is the airway: • Patent (i.e. conscious, vocalising) • At risk • Obstructed	• Suction if indicated • Head positioning • Oropharyngeal airway • Reassess • Summon expert help
B Breathing adequacy	Note/observe/perform: • Conscious level • Air movement (look, listen, feel) • Respiratory rate • Chest expansion • Use of accessory muscles/recessions • Palpation • Percussion • Auscultation • SpO_2 and FiO_2	• Administer high-flow oxygen appropriately • Support breathing with bag-mask ventilation (BMV) as necessary • Reassess • Summon expert help
C Circulation adequacy	Note/observe/perform: • Evidence of haemorrhage/fluid loss • Conscious level • Heart rate • Capillary refill time • Presence of distal/central pulses • Pulse volume features • Skin temperature and colour • Blood pressure • Urine output	• Control any external bleeding • Attach monitoring (as appropriate to setting) • Obtain circulatory access (IV or IO) • Estimate weight • Blood samples for laboratory testing and bedside glucose estimation • Fluid bolus (10–20 mL kg^{-1}) • Reassess • Summon expert help
D Disability (conscious level)	Note: • AVPU score • Interaction with parent and surroundings • Posture and muscle tone • Pupil size and reactivity	• Reconsider A, B and C management as conscious level dictates • Establish bedside glucose estimation • Establish if any medications have been given/possibly ingested • Reassess • Summon expert help
E Exposure	Note/observe: • Evidence of any blood loss/skin lesions/wounds/drains/rashes etc • Core temperature	• Reconsider specific management e.g. antibiotics in sepsis • Consider appropriate temperature control measures • Reassess • Summon expert help

My key take-home messages from this chapter

O'Driscoll BR, Howard LS, Davison AG. BTS guideline for emergency oxygen use in adult patients. Thorax 2008;63 Suppl 6:vi1-68.

Seguin P, Le Rouzo A, Tanguy M, Guillou YM, Feuillu A, Malledant Y. Evidence for the need of bedside accuracy of pylse oximetry in an intensive care unit. Critical care medicine 2000;28:703-6.

Van de Louw A, Cracco C, Cerf C, et al. Accuracy of pulse oximetry in the intensive care unit. Intensive care medicine 2001;27:1606-13.

Further reading

Brierley J, Carcillo JA, Choong K, Cornell Tet al. Clinical practice parameters for hemodynamic support of pediatric and neonatal septic shock: 2007 update from the American College of Critical Care Medicine. Critical Care Medicine 2009; 37(2):666-688.

Carcillo JA. Pediatric septic shock and multiple organ failure. Crit Care Clin 2003; 19:413-40.

De Man SA, Andre JL, Bachmann H et al. Blood pressure in childhood: pooled findings of six European studies. J Hypertension. 1991; 9:109-114.

de Oliveira CF, de Oliveira DS, Gottschald AF, et al. ACCM/PALS haemodynamic support guidelines for paediatric septic shock: an outcomes comparison with and without monitoring central venous oxygen saturation. Intensive Care Med 2008;34:1065–75.

Fleming S, Thompson M, Stevens R, et al. Normal ranges of heart rate and respiratoty rate in children from birth to 18 years of age: a systematic review of observational studies. Lancet 2011;377:1011-8.

Egdell P, Finlay L, Pedley DK. The PAWS score: validation of an early warning scoring system for the initial assessment of children in the emergency department. EMJ 2008; 25:745-9.

Lafey JG, Kavanagh BP. Hypocapnia. N Engl J Med. 2002; 347:43-53.

Levin DL, Morriss F. Essentials of Pediatric Intensive Care. Quality Medical Publishing, St. Louis, USA, 1990.

Parshuram CS, Hutchison J, Middaugh K. Development and initial validation of the bedside Paediatric Early Warning Sysytem and score. Critical Care 2009;13:R135.

Plum F, PosnerJB. The diagnostic of stupor and coma, 3rd edition. FA Davis Co, Philadelphia, USA, 1982.

Pollack MM, Fields AI, Rutimann UE et al. Sequential cardiopulmonary variables in pediatric survivors and nonsurvivors of septic shock. Crit Care Med. 1984; 12:554-559.

Basic Life Support

Contents

- Age definitions
- Infant and child basic life support sequence
- Recognition and management of choking
- Recovery positions

Learning outcomes

To enable you to:

- **Understand the importance of early effective basic life support (BLS) for decreasing mortality and morbidity**
- **Describe how and when to activate the Emergency Medical Service (EMS) or the in-hospital clinical emergency team**
- **Understand the rationale for the sequence of steps in BLS**
- **Consider the importance of early appropriate choking management**
- **Understand the rationale for the different techniques of BLS employed in infants and children**

Age definitions

For the purposes of basic life support (BLS), an infant is a baby less than one year and a child is aged between one year and puberty. It is neither appropriate nor necessary to formally establish the onset of puberty; if the rescuer thinks the victim is a child, they should use the paediatric guidelines.

Introduction

BLS is the combination of manoeuvres and skills that, without the use of technical adjuncts, provides recognition and management of a person in cardiac or respiratory arrest and 'buys time' until the victim can receive more advanced treatment.

BLS must be started as rapidly as possible. Its main objective is to achieve sufficient oxygenation and perfusion to 'protect' the brain and other vital organs. Ideally, all citizens should possess BLS knowledge and skills. The sequence of actions in BLS is known as cardiopulmonary resuscitation (CPR). BLS is more effective when the rescuer is proficient in its delivery, but even suboptimal CPR gives a better result than no CPR at all. Hence rescuers unable or unwilling to provide mouth-to-mouth ventilation should be encouraged to perform at least compression-only CPR.

BLS can be undertaken without any adjuncts; however expired air ventilation provides only 16–17% of oxygen. Oxygen should be given as soon as possible. The trained healthcare provider must provide bag-mask ventilation (BMV) with oxygen as soon as the necessary equipment is available.

Background

In the management of the collapsed child, a number of factors are critical in maximising the chances of a good outcome. The most important is the early recognition and appropriate intervention in children who exhibit signs of respiratory and/or circulatory compromise. Prevention of cardiorespiratory arrest by the optimal management of respiratory distress and/or circulatory failure will improve the prognosis (Chapter 1).

Nevertheless, there will always be some children in whom respiratory and/or circulatory collapse cannot be prevented. For these children, early BLS, rapid activation of the Emergency Medical Service (EMS) or in-hospital clinical emergency team, and prompt, effective advanced life support are crucial in improving mortality and morbidity.

BLS sequence

Although unusual, primary cardiac arrest in ventricular fibrillation (VF) or pulseless ventricular tachycardia (pVT) does occasionally occur in children. If this situation is likely, such as with the sudden, witnessed collapse of a child with a known cardiac condition, optimal outcome will depend on early defibrillation. It is then preferable for a lone rescuer to activate the EMS before starting BLS and to use an automated external defibrillator (AED), if available.

However, for the majority of children who suffer cardiorespiratory arrest, the recommended sequence of events is based on two facts:

1. Cardiorespiratory arrest is hypoxic in origin and therefore the priority is prompt oxygenation (provided by rescue breaths).

2. The most common cardiac arrhythmia is profound bradycardia deteriorating into asystole; hence effective BLS is more important than access to a defibrillator.

It is important that rescuers follow the specific order of steps in BLS because if one manoeuvre is missed or incorrectly performed, the effectiveness of the next step is likely to also be compromised.

Rescuers who have been taught adult BLS, and have no specific knowledge of paediatric resuscitation, should use the adult sequence. The following modifications ("paediatric modifiers") to the adult sequence will make it more suitable for use in children:

- Give five initial rescue breaths before starting chest compression.

- If you are on your own, perform CPR for 1 min before going for help.

- Compress the chest by at least one-third of its depth, approximately 4 cm for an infant and approximately 5 cm for an older child. Use two fingers for an infant under one year; use one or two hands for a child over one year as needed to achieve an adequate depth of compression.

Those with a duty to respond to paediatric emergencies (usually healthcare professional teams) should use the following sequence (Figure 3.1 and Figure 3.2):

S	**Safety**
S	**Stimulate**
S	**Shout for assistance**
A	**Airway**
B	**Breathing**
C	**Circulation**
R	**Reassess**

Figure 3.1 BLS sequence

S – Safety

In all emergencies quickly assess the situation and ensure the safety of first the rescuer(s) and then that of the child; although the potential hazards may be different, this is equally important whether the situation occurs within or outside the healthcare environment.

All bodily fluids should be treated as potentially infectious; put on gloves as soon as practicable and use barrier devices for ventilation (e.g. pocket mask) if possible. Whilst the efficacy of face shields is uncertain and they may not reliably prevent transmission of infection, their use affords some protection and may make it more acceptable for the receipt or delivery of rescue breaths.

On approaching the child, and before touching them, rapidly look for any clues as to what may have caused the emergency as this may influence the way the child is managed (e.g. any suspicion of head or neck injury necessitates consideration of cervical spine immobilisation).

S – Stimulate

It is important to establish the responsiveness of the apparently unconscious child by tactile and verbal stimulation as they may not be in a critical condition. You can do this by stabilising the child's head by placing one hand on their forehead and then tugging their hair, whilst calling their name or telling them to "wake up". Never shake a child vigorously.

If the child responds (e.g. moves, cries or talks), his clinical status and any further potential dangers should be assessed, and if necessary, help obtained.

If there is no response continue with BLS as described below.

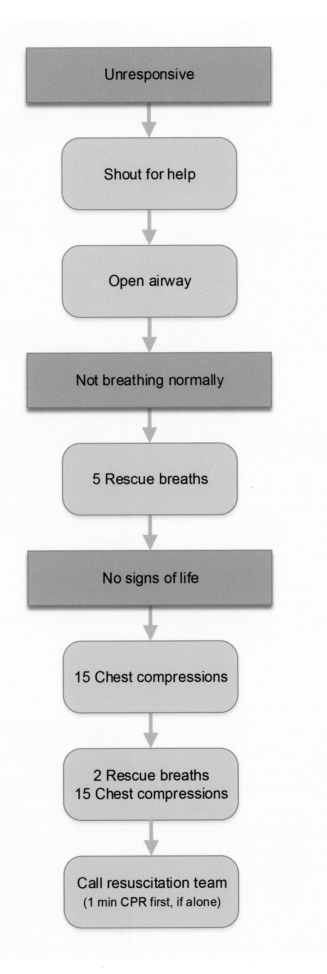

Figure 3.2 Paediatric BLS algorithm G2015

S – Shout

If there is only one rescuer, they must not leave the child (or delay BLS to use a mobile telephone), but shout "help" as they start BLS. If there is another person present, they should be asked to summon the emergency medical services (EMS).

This second rescuer should get help by dialling 999 or 112 for the EMS if out-of-hospital, or 2222 for the hospital clinical emergency team. They must be able to convey the specific information listed in Table 3.1.

Table 3.1 Information required when requesting EMS	
National 999 or 112 ambulance request	**In-hospital 2222 request**
Precise location of the emergency	Precise location of the emergency
Type of emergency (e.g. infant in cardiorespiratory arrest, child in road traffic accident)	Specific clinical emergency team required (e.g. paediatric, paediatric trauma)
Number and age of victim(s)	Any other local policy requirements
Severity and urgency of the situation	

The caller should only end the phone call once the operator confirms no further information is needed. They should then return to the rescuer(s) delivering BLS and inform them that the EMS has been activated. If the event is within a healthcare environment, appropriate clinical emergency equipment should also be taken to the patient.

A – Airway

In the unconscious child, the tongue is likely to at least partly occlude their airway. This can usually be overcome by using a head tilt and chin lift manoeuvre or, if necessary, by performing a jaw thrust.

Head tilt and chin lift

This is a simple and effective initial manoeuvre. To perform the head tilt, approach the child from the side, place one hand on their forehead and gently tilt their head back. In infants, the head should be placed in a neutral position (Figure 3.3). For the child, a 'sniffing' position that causes some extension of the head on the neck will be required (Figure 3.4).

The chin lift is performed by placing the fingertips of the rescuer's other hand on the bony part of the child's lower jaw, and lifting the chin upwards. Take care not to compress the soft tissues under the child's jaw as this will occlude the airway.

Jaw thrust

This is the preferred airway opening manoeuvre when cervical spine immobilisation is required. To perform a jaw

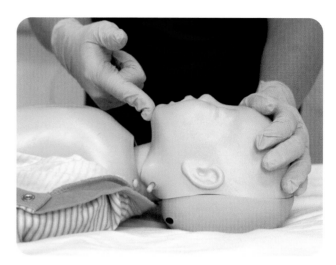

Figure 3.3 Head tilt and chin lift in an infant (neutral position)

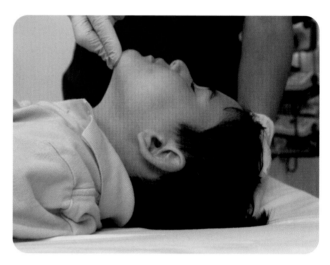

Figure 3.4 Head tilt and chin lift in a child ('sniffing position)

thrust, approach the child from behind and place hands on either side of the child's head. Two or three fingertips of both hands should be placed under both angles of the child's lower jaw. With thumbs resting gently on the child's cheeks, lift the jaw upwards. The rescuers elbows should rest on the surface that the child is laid on (Figure 3.5).

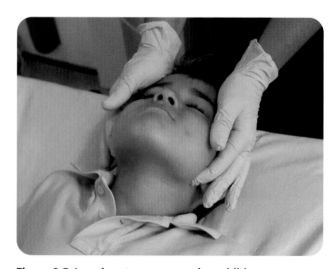

Figure 3.5 Jaw thrust manoeuvre in a child

Whichever method of airway opening is used, a brief check can be made to ensure there is no obvious foreign body present. If a foreign body is seen and the rescuer is confident that they can remove it, easily, this can be done, but blind finger sweeps should never be performed. The management of choking is discussed later in this chapter.

B – Breathing

Assessing for normal breathing

After opening the airway, the rescuer needs to assess the child for effective, normal breathing. The best way to do this is to 'look, listen and feel' whilst maintaining the airway opening manoeuvre.

LOOK	for chest (and abdominal) movements
LISTEN	for airflow at the mouth and nose (+/- additional noises)
FEEL	for airflow at the mouth and nose

The rescuer positions themselves with their cheek just a few centimetres above the child's mouth and nose, and looks along the child's chest for no more than 10 s (Figures 3.6 and 3.7).

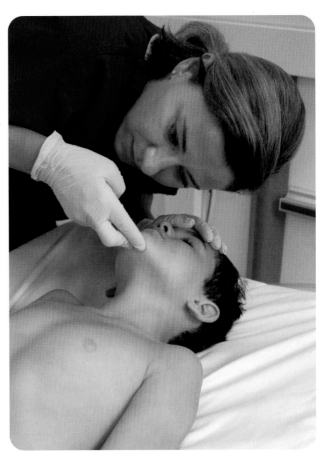

Figure 3.7 Checking for breathing in a child

If the child is breathing normally and effectively, maintain the airway opening manoeuvre whilst help is summoned; however, if there is no-one else to activate the EMS, the rescuer must do this themselves. Unless contraindicated (i.e. suspicion of spinal injury) the child should be placed in a safe side-lying position (described later in this chapter) until further help arrives.

If the child is not breathing normally, or they are only gasping ineffectively (agonal breathing), the rescuer must immediately attempt five rescue breaths. Agonal breathing is infrequent or irregular, noisy gasps, which must not be confused with normal breathing.

Delivery of expired air rescue breaths

The aim of rescue breaths is to deliver oxygen to the child's lungs. Until an appropriate ventilation device is available, expired air rescue breathing is required. This will provide approximately 16–17% oxygen. The effectiveness of rescue breaths is assessed by observing the rise and fall of the child's chest wall; rescuers may need to adapt the pressure and volume of breath delivery to the individual child to ensure that chest movement is obtained with each breath delivered.

Five initial rescue breaths should be attempted. Each breath should be delivered slowly (over approximately 1 s). This maximises the amount of oxygen delivered to the child's lungs and minimises the risk of gastric distension. By inhaling deeply themselves between each rescue

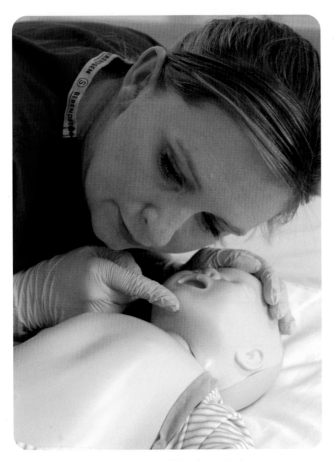

Figure 3.6 Checking for breathing in an infant

breath, the rescuer can optimise the oxygen and minimise the amount of carbon dioxide they deliver to the child. The effectiveness of the rescue breaths can only be determined by observing the rise and fall of the chest. The rescuer must adapt the pressure and volume of inhalation to the characteristics of the child to ensure that chest movement is seen with each breath given.

If chest movement is not observed with attempted delivery of a rescue breath, reassess the child's airway (i.e. reposition the child's head) and ensure there is an adequate seal between their mouth and the child's face before attempting the next breath. If, despite repositioning the child's head and having an adequate seal, the rescuer is still unable to achieve movement of the child's chest after five attempts, the likelihood of choking should be considered and the rescuer should move straight to chest compressions.

Mouth-to-mouth and nose rescue breathing

This is the recommended technique for giving expired air rescue breaths to an infant. The rescuer places their mouth around both the mouth and nose to create a tight seal, and then blows into the infant (Figure 3.8). If it is not possible to cover both the mouth and nose, blow into either the infant's mouth or nose (with the nostrils occluded or the mouth closed, to minimise escape of air).

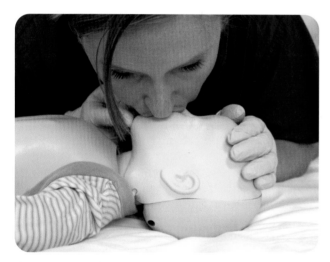

Figure 3.8 Mouth-to-mouth and nose rescue breath delivery in an infant

Mouth-to-mouth rescue breathing

This is the recommended technique for giving expired air rescue breaths to a child. The rescuer places their mouth over the child's mouth, creating a seal. Using the fingers of their hand at the top of the child's head, the rescuer occludes the child's nostrils to ensure that the rescue breath does not escape through the child's nose (Figure 3.9).

C – Circulation

Assessing for 'signs of life'

After the five initial rescue breaths attempts are given, determine whether the child has an adequate

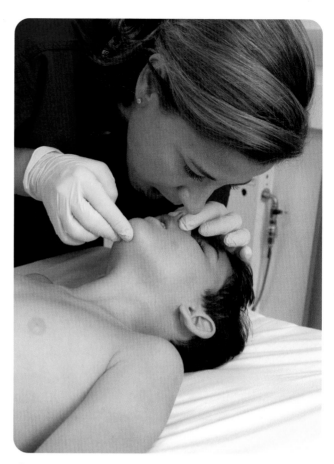

Figure 3.9 Mouth-to-mouth rescue breath delivery in a child

spontaneous circulation, or if they also require chest compressions. The time taken to assess the circulation should **not exceed 10 s.** Observe the child for signs of life.

Signs of life include:

- **swallowing**
- **vocalising**
- **coughing**
- **normal (not agonal) breathing**

For healthcare professionals who are trained in pulse checking, a central pulse can be palpated, whilst simultaneously looking for 'signs of life'.

In infants the recommended sites for central pulse palpation are the femoral or brachial artery (Figure 3.10). In the child it is the femoral or carotid artery (Figure 3.11).

If there are no 'signs of life', chest compressions should be started immediately, unless the rescuer is **certain** they can feel a definite pulse > 60 min⁻¹ **within 10 s.** If there is any doubt, start chest compressions.

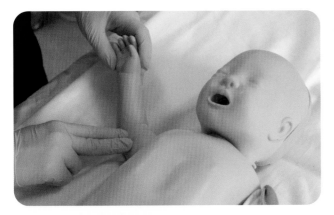

Figure 3.10 Brachial pulse palpation on an infant

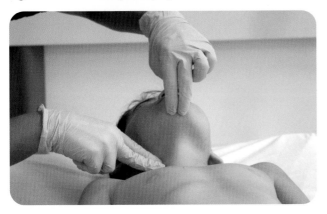

Figure 3.11 Carotid pulse palpation on a child

If there are 'signs of life' and/or a pulse is found (i.e. > 60 min^{-1}), reassess the child's breathing. If breathing is absent or inadequate (e.g. agonal breathing) then rescue breathing should be continued at a rate of 12–20 breaths min^{-1}. The child's breathing and circulation should be frequently reassessed and BLS continued until either the EMS arrives to take over, or until the child starts to breathe spontaneously.

If effective spontaneous breathing is established, and there is no suspicion of cervical spine trauma, the child should be placed in a safe, side-lying position.

Principles of chest compressions

Chest compressions are serial, rhythmic compressions of the anterior chest wall, intended to cause blood to flow to vital organ tissues in an attempt to keep them viable until return of spontaneous circulation (ROSC) is achieved.

The recommended ratio of chest compressions to ventilations for infants and children is 15:2. However, a lone healthcare professional may choose to use the standard adult ratio of 30:2 to avoid changing frequently between rescue breathing and chest compression. For simplicity, lay persons are taught to use the adult 30:2 ratio. Whichever ratio is used, chest compressions must be performed effectively and to a high quality to achieve the best outcomes.

The rate of chest compressions should be 100–120 min^{-1}; it should be noted that when interspersed with rescue breaths, the actual number of compressions delivered will be less than this.

Effective chest compression is facilitated by ensuring the child or infant is lying on a firm flat surface. It requires depression of the infant's chest by approximately 4 cm and the child's chest by approximately 5 cm with equal time spent in the compression and relaxation phases.

During the relaxation phase of each compression, fully release the pressure whilst leaving the hand(s)/fingers in position on the child's chest wall.

At the end of each series of chest compressions, the hand(s)/fingers must be removed from the child's chest in order to effectively perform airway opening manoeuvres and give two rescue breaths.

Resuscitation Council (UK), ERC and AHA guidelines indicate that the following are important in order to deliver high quality CPR:

1. Chest compression fraction (the % of time during resuscitation spent delivering chest compressions, CCF) > 80%
2. Depth of chest compressions – infants 4 cm, children 5cm
3. Rate of chest compressions – all ages 100–120 chest compressions (CC) per minute
4. No lean – allow full chest recoil
5. Ventilation rate –10 –12 breaths per minute all ages

Landmarking for chest compressions

In all infants and children, deliver chest compressions over the lower half of the sternum. In order to avoid compressing the upper abdomen, locate the xiphisternum at the angle where the lower costal margins meet and compress one finger's breadth above this point (Figure 3.12).

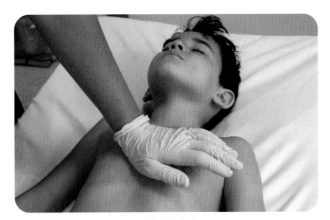

Figure 3.12 Landmarking for chest compressions on a child

Performing chest compressions

Infant chest compression

Two-finger technique

This is the recommended method of infant chest compression for the lone rescuer. Having landmarked as described above, place two fingers of one hand in the correct position on the sternum and depress it by 4 cm (at least one third of the anteroposterior diameter) (Figure 3.13 and Figure 3.14).

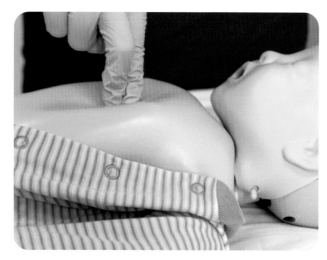

Figure 3.13 Two-finger chest compression on an infant – depression phase

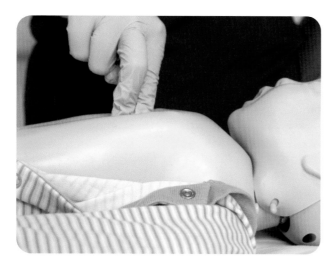

Figure 3.14 Two-finger chest compression on an infant – relaxation phase

Two-thumb encircling technique

This is the recommended method of infant chest compression for two rescuers. There is evidence that this method delivers greater cardiac output than the two-finger technique, but it is difficult for a single rescuer to perform and also deliver timely and effective rescue breaths. It is therefore usually reserved for in-hospital resuscitation where there are two rescuers and ventilation delivery devices can be used.

The two-thumb encircling technique requires a healthcare professional to be positioned at the infant's head to maintain the airway and deliver ventilation. A second rescuer, at the infant's side (or at their feet), places their two thumbs side-by-side in the correct position on the lower half of the sternum (Figure 3.15). In a very small baby, the thumbs may be placed one on top of the other. The rest of the rescuer's hands are then able to support the infant's back as they encircle the chest wall. Chest compressions are delivered as described previously, it is very important to allow full chest recoil with this method.

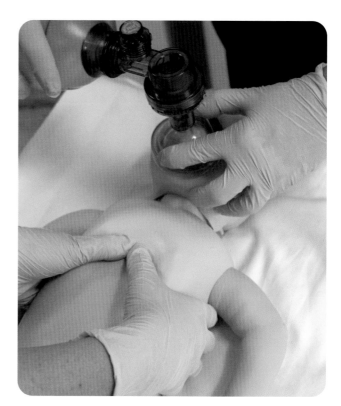

Figure 3.15 Two-thumb encircling chest compressions on an infant

Child chest compression

Having landmarked as previously described, the rescuer should position themselves at one side of the child, and place the heel of one hand along the long axis of the lower half of the child's sternum. The fingers should be raised off the chest so that pressure is exerted only through the heel of the hand and on to the sternum.

By positioning themselves so that their elbow is locked straight, and their shoulders are directly over the heel of their hand on the child's chest, the rescuer can use their body weight to depress the sternum by 5 cm (at least one third of the anteroposterior diameter). In larger children or for small rescuers, this is achieved more effectively by using both hands with the fingers interlocked together off the chest wall (Figure 3.16).

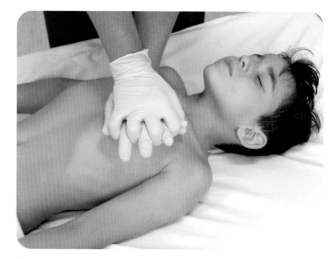

Figure 3.16 Two-handed chest compression on a child

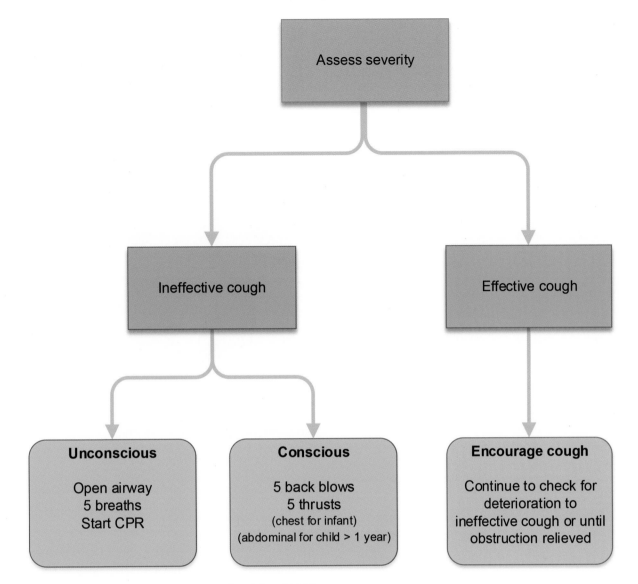

Figure 3.17 Paediatric choking treatment algorithm G2015

R – Reassess

After approximately one minute of BLS, a single rescuer should stop to go and call the EMS unless a second person was available to do this. Use a mobile phone if available. Otherwise, if the victim is an infant or a very small child, the rescuer may be able to carry him safely to activate a telephone to summon further assistance, and then continue CPR. If the child is too large to carry, leave the child to activate the EMS, and return to recommence BLS as soon as possible.

If the EMS has already been activated, the rescuer should immediately resume BLS unless there are obvious 'signs of life'.

Continuation of BLS

BLS should only be stopped when:

- the child exhibits adequate 'signs of life'

- further rescuers take over resuscitation

- the single rescuer is too exhausted to continue.

As soon as the EMS and/or appropriate paediatric resuscitation equipment becomes available, advanced life support techniques can start.

Choking

When a foreign body enters their airway, a child will react immediately by coughing in an attempt to expel it. A child who is choking on a foreign body but is still able to cough effectively must be actively encouraged to do so. A spontaneous cough is not only safer, but it is probably more effective than any manoeuvre a rescuer might perform.

However, if coughing is absent or becoming ineffective, the child's airway is at risk of complete obstruction, which will rapidly result in asphyxiation. Any child, who is unable to effectively cough as a result of foreign body aspiration, requires immediate interventions (Figure 3.17).

Recognition of choking

Choking is characterised by the sudden onset of respiratory distress associated with coughing, gagging or stridor.

The majority of choking events in infants and children occur during play or feeding, and are therefore frequently witnessed by an adult which means interventions can start immediately. However, it is important to be aware that the signs of choking (Table 3.2) can be confused with those of other causes of airway obstruction (e.g. laryngitis or epiglottitis), which require different management.

Table 3.2 Signs of choking

General signs
Witnessed episode
Coughing or choking
Sudden onset
Recent history of playing with, or eating small objects

Ineffective cough	Effective cough
Unable to vocalise	Crying or verbal response to questions
Quiet or silent cough	
Unable to breathe	Loud cough
Cyanosis	Able to take a breath before coughing
Decreasing level of consciousness	Fully responsive

Management of choking

If the child is coughing effectively, no external manoeuvre is necessary. Encourage the child to cough and observe them closely.

If the child's coughing is absent or becoming ineffective, shout for help and quickly determine the child's conscious level.

Conscious infants and children

If the child is conscious but their coughing is absent or ineffective, deliver back blows. These are intended to loosen the object for the child to be able to then expel it. If back blows do not relieve the airway obstruction, thrusts should be given; chest thrusts for infants and abdominal thrusts for children. These thrusts are intended as an 'artificial cough'; they increase the intrathoracic pressure which will facilitate expulsion of the foreign body.

Delivery of back blows to an infant

1. To deliver back blows safely, sit on a chair or kneel on the floor, and hold the infant in a head downwards, prone position across their lap (Figure 3.18).

2. Support the infant's head by placing the thumb of one hand at the angle of the lower jaw, and one or two fingers from the same hand at the same point on the other side of the infant's face. Care must be taken not to compress the soft tissues under the infant's jaw.

3. Up to five sharp back blows should be delivered to the middle of the infant's back, between their scapulae, with the heel of the other hand.

The aim is to relieve the obstruction with each individual back blow rather than to give all five.

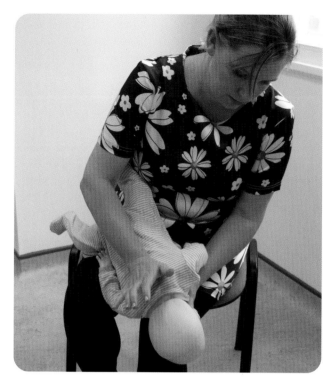

Figure 3.18 Delivery of back blows to an infant

Delivery of back blows to a child

1. To maximise effectiveness, try to support the child in a head downwards position (Figure 3.19). If the child is too large to do this safely, they should be supported in a forward-leaning position, with the rescuer delivering the back blows from behind.

2. Up to five sharp back blows should be delivered to the middle of the child's back, between their scapulae, with the heel of the rescuer's other hand.

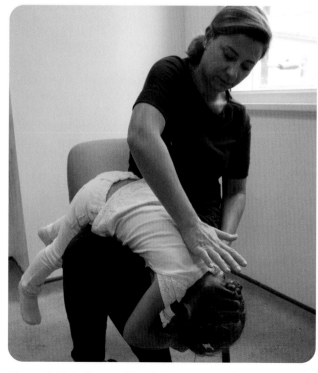

Figure 3.19 Delivery of back blows to a child

The aim is to relieve the obstruction with each individual back blow rather than to give all five.

If back blows fail to dislodge the foreign body and the infant/child is still conscious, deliver thrusts. In infants these are delivered to the chest, and are similar to chest compressions. However, in children over one year, abdominal thrusts may be performed. If the clinical judgement is that the child is too small to tolerate abdominal thrusts, then chest thrusts can be delivered instead. **Abdominal thrusts (Heimlich manoeuvre) must not be performed on infants.**

Delivery of chest thrusts to an infant

1. Turn the infant from the head down, prone position they were in for back blow delivery, into a head downwards, supine position. This can be safely achieved by placement of the rescuer's free arm along the infant's back, with the hand encircling the infant's occiput. The infant should then be turned over whilst keeping his head lower than his trunk.

2. The rescuer supports the infant down along their arm which is supported down or across their thigh.

3. The landmark for chest compressions should be identified on the infant's sternum and up to five sharp downward thrusts delivered. These thrusts are similar to chest compressions but they are sharper in nature and delivered at a slower rate.

The aim is to relieve the obstruction with each individual chest thrust rather than to give all five.

Delivery of abdominal thrusts to a child over one year

1. To maximise safety, the rescuer should stand behind the child, and support them in a forward leaning position by placing their arms underneath the child's and encircling their torso.

2. The rescuer should clench one of their fists and place it against the child's abdomen, approximately midway between the umbilicus and the xiphisternum.

3. By grasping their fist with their free hand, the rescuer should deliver the abdominal thrusts by pulling sharply inwards and upwards up to five times (Figure 3.20). Care should be taken not to exert pressure over the xiphoid process or the lower rib cage as this may result in thoracic or intra-abdominal trauma.

The aim is to relieve the obstruction with each individual abdominal thrust rather than to give all five.

Reassessment

Following delivery of the chest or abdominal thrusts, reassess the child.

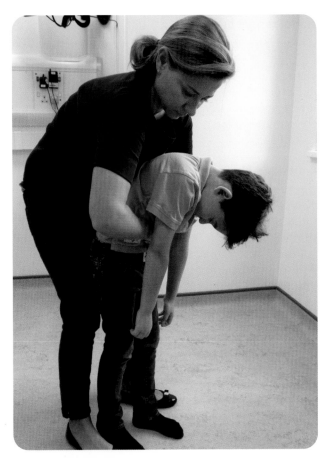

Figure 3.20 Delivery of abdominal thrusts to a child

If the foreign body has been successfully expelled, the child may still need medical assistance; a piece of the object may remain in the respiratory tract and cause further complications. As abdominal thrusts can cause injury, a child who has received them should be examined by a medical practitioner.

If the foreign body has not been expelled and the child remains conscious, repeat the sequence of back blows and thrusts as indicated. Do not leave the child at this stage, but call out again to ensure that the EMS has been called.

Unresponsive infants and children

If the child is, or becomes, unconscious from choking, they should be placed supine on a firm, flat surface, whilst the rescuer shouts for help. If, a second rescuer is available, they should be sent to activate the EMS. If there is only one rescuer, they must not leave the child at this stage, but proceed with BLS as described earlier in this chapter, with particular attention to the following points:

Checking the mouth

Each time the airway is opened for rescue breaths, look to see if they can detect the foreign body in the child's mouth. If it is visible, a single finger sweep can be attempted to remove the object. However, blind or repeated finger sweeps must not be performed as these are likely to impact the object further down the pharynx and/or cause trauma.

Initial rescue breaths

When a rescue breath attempt does not result in chest wall expansion, the child's head should be repositioned before attempting the next breath. If, despite repositioning, all five rescue breaths are ineffective and the child remains unresponsive (no 'signs of life'), proceed straight to chest compressions without further assessment of the circulation.

Continued BLS

Continue with BLS for approximately one minute, or five cycles of 15 compressions to 2 ventilations before summoning the EMS (if this has not already been done by someone else).

If the child displays signs of life, the rescuer should assess their ABC and continue as appropriate.

Recovery positions

Unless contraindicated, the unresponsive child who has effective spontaneous breathing should be placed in a safe side-lying position (Figure 3.21).

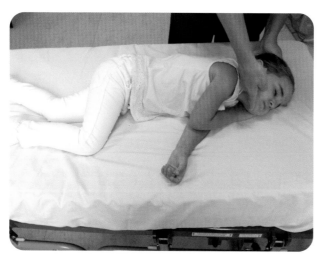

Figure 3.21 An unresponsive child in a safe side-lying position

The purpose of placing an unresponsive child in such a position is to ensure that their tongue does not fall backwards occluding their pharynx, and to reduce the potential risk of aspiration should they vomit.

There is no universally accepted 'recovery' position for children, but there are general principles to be considered when placing the child in a safe position. These include ensuring that the child:

- has a patent airway

- can drain secretions/vomit freely from their mouth

- is in a stable position that they cannot easily roll over from (this may require the placement of a rolled-up towel or blanket behind their back in small infants)

- can be easily observed

- can be easily turned on to their back if they require resuscitation interventions

- is in as near a true lateral position as possible

- has no pressure on their chest that may impede breathing

If the child needs to be in this position for longer than an hour, they should be turned on to their other side to relieve the pressure on the lower arm.

Summary learning

- **Always ensure safety before undertaking BLS.**

- **The preferred ratio of chest compressions: ventilations is 15:2 when BLS is being delivered by healthcare professionals but in some instances it may be appropriate to adopt the standard adult 30:2 sequence.**

- **One full minute of BLS should be performed by lone rescuers before they activate EMS (except on the rare occasion that a primary cardiac arrest is suspected).**

- **Management of conscious choking infants consists of back blows followed by chest thrusts.**

- **Management of conscious choking children consists of back blows followed by abdominal thrusts.**

- **Management of unconscious infants and children with choking requires BLS to be performed.**

My key take-home messages from this chapter

EPALS

Further reading

Atkins DL, Everson-Stewart S, Sears GK, Daya M, Osmond MH, Warden CR, et al. Epidemiology and outcomes from out-of-hospital cardiac arrest in children: the Resuscitation Outcomes Consortium Epistry-Cardiac Arrest. Circulation. 2009 Mar 24;119(11):1484-91.

Nadkarni VM, Larkin GL, Peberdy MA, Carey SM, Kaye W, Mancini ME, et al. First documented rhythm and clinical outcome from in-hospital cardiac arrest among children and adults. JAMA. 2006 Jan 4;295(1):50-7.

Kitamura T, Iwami T, Kawamura T, Nagao K, Tanaka H, Nadkarni VM, et al. Conventional and chest-compression-only cardiopulmonary resuscitation by bystanders for children who have out-of-hospital cardiac arrests: a prospective, nationwide, population-based cohort study. Lancet. 2010 Apr 17;375(9723):1347-54.

Kao PC, Chiang WC, Yang CW, Chen SJ, Liu YP, Lee CC, et al. What is the correct depth of chest compression for infants and children? A radiological study. Pediatrics. 2009 Jul;124(1):49-55.

Meyer A, Nadkarni V, Pollock A, Babbs C, Nishisaki A, Braga M, et al. Evaluation of the Neonatal Resuscitation Program's recommended chest compression depth using computerized tomography imaging. Resuscitation. 2010 May;81(5):544-8.

Sutton RM, Niles D, Nysaether J, Arbogast KB, Nishisaki A, Maltese MR, et al. Pediatric CPR quality monitoring: analysis of thoracic anthropometric data. Resuscitation. 2009 Oct;80(10):1137-41.

Babbs SF, Nadkarni V. Optimizing chest compression to rescue ventilation ratios during one-rescue CPR by professionals and laypersons: children are not just little adults. Resuscitation 2004; 61:173-81.

Berg RA, Hilwig RW et al. "Simulated mouth-to-mouth ventilation and chest compressions (bystander cardiopulmonary resuscitation) improves outcome in a swine model of prehospital pediatric asphyxial cardiac arrest." Crit Care Med 1999; 27(9):1893-1899.

Berg RA, Hilwig RW et al. "Bystander" chest compressions and assisted ventilation independently improve outcome from piglet asphyxial pulseless "cardiac arrest". Circulation 2000; 101(14):1743-1748.

Tibballs J, Russell P. Reliability of pulse palpation by healthcare personnel to diagnose paediatric cardiac arrest. Resuscitation. 2009 Jan;80(1):61-4.

EPALS

Advanced management of the airway and ventilation

Contents

- Airway management using positioning and adjuncts
- Oxygen delivery devices
- Assisted ventilation methods
- Supraglottic airway (SGA) devices, intubation and capnography

Learning outcomes

To enable you to:

- Recognise upper airway obstruction
- Discuss methods used to open the airway during initial resuscitation
- Consider the use of oxygen delivery systems during initial resuscitation
- Describe the methods used to assist ventilation during initial resuscitation
- Understand the role of advanced airways (laryngeal masks and tracheal tubes)

As previously described, the most common cause of cardiorespiratory arrest in children is secondary to respiratory failure resulting in hypoxia and acidosis. The outcome is poor following hypoxic induced cardiorespiratory arrest, therefore the management of the airway and ventilation (breathing) is the first priority in dealing with the seriously ill child regardless of the underlying cause. Early recognition and adequate management of compensated respiratory failure are essential. This chapter describes the initial advanced management of the airway and ventilation based on the child's physiological dysfunction.

Airway obstruction

Airway obstruction is a common occurrence in the seriously ill child. It may be the primary cause of the cardiorespiratory arrest (e.g. choking) or a consequence of the underlying disease process (i.e. hypoxia), which leads to loss of consciousness. In the unconscious child, the tongue can fall backwards and occlude their airway (Figure 4.1). Regardless of the cause, airway obstruction must be rapidly recognised and managed to prevent secondary hypoxic damage to the vital organs.

Recognition of airway obstruction

In a conscious child, airway obstruction may be demonstrated by difficulty in breathing and/or increased respiratory effort. In both conscious and unconscious children, there may be additional respiratory noises if the obstruction is partial, whereas respiration will be silent if there is complete obstruction.

The most effective way to detect airway obstruction in all children is to look, listen and feel.

EPALS

LOOK	for chest (and abdominal) movements
LISTEN	for airflow at the mouth and nose (+/- additional noises)
FEEL	for airflow at the mouth and nose

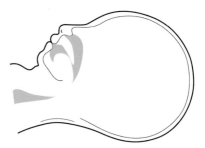

Figure 4.1 Unconscious child, the tongue falls backwards and obstructs the airway

LOOK for breathing – during normal breathing, the chest wall expands and the abdomen is pushed slightly outwards as the diaphragm contracts. When the airway is obstructed however, the abdomen protrudes markedly and the chest is drawn inwards when the diaphragm contracts during inspiration ('see-saw' respiration). Additionally, accessory muscle usage and recession are likely to be observed. It can be difficult to differentiate these paradoxical movements from normal breathing, and the rescuer must also listen for the presence or absence of breath sounds and feel for air movement. If a clear facemask is being used, misting of the mask may be observed.

LISTEN for breathing – normal respiration is quiet. Partially obstructed breathing is noisy, whilst completely obstructed breathing will be silent.

FEEL for breathing – the movement of air on inspiration and expiration can be felt at the mouth and nose (or tracheostomy) during normal breathing. If there is airway obstruction this will be limited or absent.

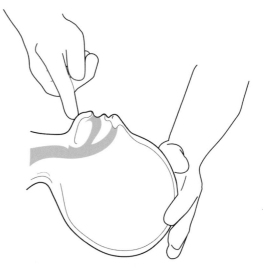

Figure 4.2 Head tilt chin lift opens the airway

Partial airway obstruction can quickly deteriorate to complete obstruction and therefore must always be considered as an emergency. Complete airway obstruction will lead to profound hypoxia, vital organ failure and cardiorespiratory arrest if the obstruction is not relieved very rapidly. Immediate action must be taken to relieve the obstruction and clear the airway.

Techniques to optimise the airway

Conscious children

If the child is making adequate spontaneous respiratory effort, they should be supported in a position of comfort (preferably the one they naturally assume themselves to optimise their airway). High flow oxygen should be given in a manner that the child will tolerate, whilst experienced help is sought.

Unconscious children

Whether or not the child is making spontaneous respiratory effort, the patency of the airway needs to be optimised immediately. This initially means positioning their head by performing either a head tilt and chin lift, or a jaw thrust manoeuvre.

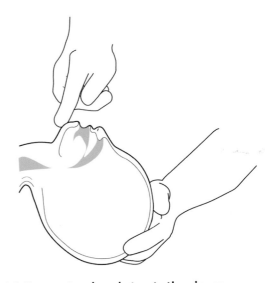

Figure 4.3 Hyperextension obstructs the airway

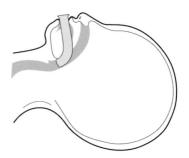

Figure 4.4 Airway adjunct keeps the tongue forward

Additionally, suction may be required to clear secretions, vomit or blood.

Head positioning

Open the child's airway by performing a head tilt and chin lift (Figure 4.2) or jaw thrust manoeuvre (Chapter 3). It is extremely important to ensure that head positioning techniques are carried out properly to make certain that neither hyperextension (Figure 4.3) nor excessive flexion of the neck occurs, as both will make obstruction worse. Take care not to compress the soft tissues under the child's jaw as this can also occlude the airway.

Suction

Standard suction devices in hospital are pipeline units. They consist of a wall terminal outlet, vacuum pressure regulator, a reservoir, tubing and a connector for an appropriate suction catheter to be attached.

In some low dependency hospital areas, during transportation and non-hospital environments such as GP surgeries, it is likely that the suction device available will be a portable device that is operated by battery or a hand/foot pump.

Large bore rigid suction catheters (e.g. Yankauer) are particularly useful for the clearance of thick or excessive secretions and vomit. Soft, flexible catheters in a range of sizes should also be available as these may be less traumatic to use and are particularly useful for nasal suction. They can also be passed through nasopharyngeal or oropharyngeal airways and tracheal tubes but they may not allow adequate clearance of thick or copious secretions.

Whichever suction catheter types are used, they should ideally have a side hole that can be occluded by the rescuer's finger to allow greater control over the suction pressure generated. Suction pressure should not exceed 120 mmHg in infants.

Airway suction must be carried out cautiously if the child has an intact gag reflex as it may induce vomiting which can lead to aspiration.

Airway opening adjuncts

Oropharyngeal airways

The oropharyngeal airway (e.g. Guedel) is a rigid curved tube that is designed to open a channel between the lips and the base of the tongue (Figure 4.4). They are made of plastic and are reinforced and flanged at the proximal end. Available sizes range from 000 for premature infants to 4–5 for large adults (Figure 4.5).

The correctly sized airway is one that, when laid against the side of the face, has a length equal to the distance between the level of the patient's incisors (or where they will be) to the angle of their jaw (Figure 4.6). If an incorrect

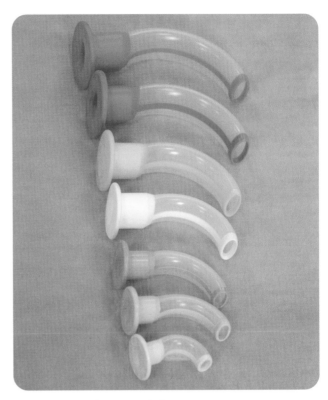

Figure 4.5 Oropharyngeal airways

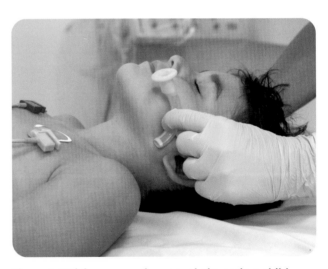

Figure 4.6 Sizing an oropharyngeal airway in a child

size is used, it may result in trauma, laryngospasm and/or worsening of the airway obstruction.

The oropharyngeal airway should be inserted with great care using the minimum of force to avoid trauma and bleeding of the delicate palatal and pharyngeal mucosa. It is important to ensure that the tip of the oropharyngeal airway does not push the tongue back into the pharynx.

The airway can be introduced directly, sliding it carefully over the tongue or alternatively, it can be introduced upside down initially, as follows:

- place the tip with the concave side of the airway facing the roof of the mouth

- insert the airway past the teeth and gums pushing the tongue away from the roof of the mouth with the convex side of the airway

- rotate it 180° as it passes beyond the hard palate and into the oropharynx

- ensure that the flange rests over the mouth

Whichever technique is used, the effort required to insert the oropharyngeal airway should be minimal; do not use force.

Oropharyngeal airways are intended to be used in unconscious patients. If the child is semi-conscious they may cough, gag, vomit or develop laryngospasm. Insertion of the oropharyngeal airway should be abandoned if this occurs.

Following insertion of the oropharyngeal airway, the child's airway patency should be reassessed by the 'look, listen and feel' approach and oxygen given if indicated.

Nasopharyngeal airways

The nasopharyngeal airway is a flexible tube that is designed to open a channel between the nostril and the nasopharynx. They are made of soft plastic or silicone, are bevelled at the insertion end and flanged at the outer end (Figure 4.7). The flange prevents the airway passing completely into the nasal passage. Tracheal tubes cut to the correct length may alternatively be used.

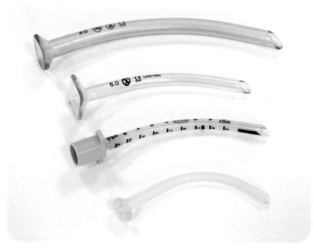

Figure 4.7 Nasopharyngeal airway

The correct insertion depth should be sized from the nostrils to the angle of the mandible. An appropriate tube size can be estimated by matching its diameter against the diameter of the child's anterior nares and when inserted it should not cause blanching of the nostril.

Once appropriately sized, the nasopharyngeal airway should be lubricated and introduced into the nostril. With a gentle rotating motion, the airway should be passed directly backwards and posteriorly along the floor of the nostril. The tube should not be directed upwards as this

will cause trauma and bleeding (Figure 4.8). Following insertion of the nasopharyngeal airway, the child's airway patency should be reassessed by the 'look, listen and feel' approach and oxygen given if indicated.

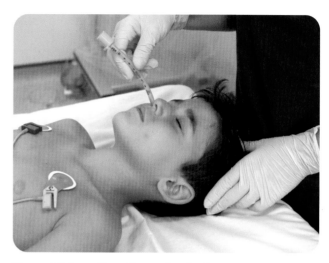

Figure 4.8 Insertion of a tracheal tube as a nasopharyngeal airway

Nasopharyngeal airways may be better tolerated by conscious children than oropharyngeal airways and are useful as adjuncts in the management of children who may improve their level of consciousness (e.g. the fitting child who is becoming less obtunded).

Their use is contraindicated in patients where basal skull fracture is suspected or if there is a coagulopathy.

Oxygen delivery systems

Oxygen should be given as soon as it is available. Initially, this should be at the highest available concentration for all seriously ill children; concerns about oxygen toxicity should never prevent its use during resuscitation. Oxygen should be regulated using a flowmeter capable of delivering up to 15 L min^{-1} (although this may be much higher when high flow nasal cannulae are used via a special flowmeter). It should ideally be warmed and humidified to minimise the risks of airway irritation and hypothermia. The method used to deliver the oxygen should be selected according to the child's clinical condition. Oxygen saturation levels should be monitored by pulse oximetry (SpO_2). When the child's condition has stabilised, the inspired oxygen concentration should be reduced, whilst monitoring SpO_2 to maintain adequate oxygenation. Table 4.1 shows the amount of oxygen that is delivered for each oxygen delivery device.

Oxygen mask with reservoir bag

This is the preferred method for delivering oxygen in the seriously ill child who is breathing spontaneously. The flow of oxygen must be sufficiently high to ensure the reservoir bag fills adequately (Figure 4.9). It is possible to give an oxygen concentration up to 90% with an oxygen delivery flow of 12–15 L min^{-1} depending on the child's minute volume (the product of the tidal volume of each breath and the number of breaths min^{-1}).

Table 4.1 Oxygen delivery devices, flow rates and maximum inspired oxygen levels

Device	Flow rate	Maximum inspired
Nasal prongs	Maximum 4 L min^{-1}	40%
Oxygen mask without reservoir	10–15 L min^{-1}	60%
Oxygen mask with reservoir	Must be enough to avoid reservoir collapse during inspiration, e.g. 12–15 L min^{-1}	90%
Bag Mask Reservoir (BMV)	15 L min^{-1}	90%
High flow nasal cannulae	2–30 L min^{-1}*	100%

*Will vary between manufacturers

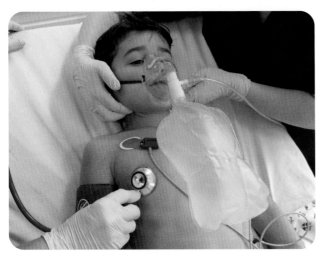

Figure 4.9 Non re-breathing oxygen mask with reservoir

These devices have three 'one-way' flap-valves; one between the oxygen supply port/reservoir bag and the mask, and one on each side of the facemask over the inspiratory holes.

The mask works as follows:

- When the child inhales, the valve between oxygen supply port/reservoir bag and the mask opens allowing oxygen to flow in to the mask, whilst the ones on either side of the mask close so reducing entrainment of room air, hence minimising the dilution of the higher concentration of inspired oxygen.

- When the child exhales, the valve between oxygen supply port/reservoir bag and the mask closes whilst the ones on either side of the mask opens to allow escape of the child's expired breath (i.e. there is no rebreathing of gas).

Note: if the flap-valves are inadvertently removed, re-breathing and dilution of inspired oxygen can occur.

Simple oxygen mask

A simple oxygen mask without a reservoir bag can deliver oxygen concentrations of up to 60% at flow rates of 10–15 L min^{-1}. Room air is entrained around the edges of the mask and through the holes in the mask so diluting the oxygen delivery.

'Blow-by' facial oxygen

Either the end of the oxygen tubing or a facemask can be held by the child's carer at a short distance from the child's face. This is a less threatening method that can help to alleviate the child's fear and maximise their cooperation. However, the inspired concentration that can be delivered is low and inconsistent, so it is only suitable for children with mild respiratory compromise who cannot tolerate other methods of oxygen delivery. Oxygen flow rates need to be adjusted depending what the child will accept.

Nasal cannulae

This method can be useful in stable children of all ages, particularly in pre-school children. The delivery of oxygen via cannulae (or 'prongs') is dependent on oxygen flow and nasal resistance but the FiO$_2$ will be low and variable, so it is not suitable during resuscitation or when a high oxygen concentration is required. They are also not suitable for use in children with copious or tenacious nasal secretions, as they will easily become blocked. Flow rates should be kept below 4 L min^{-1} as higher flows are extremely irritating to the nasal passages and do not significantly increase oxygen delivery.

High flow nasal cannula oxygen

High flow nasal cannula oxygen (e.g. optiflow) is increasingly being used for critically ill patients, as it has the advantage of humidifying and warming the gases. It is also able to deliver a higher FiO$_2$ than standard nasal cannulae. At high oxygen flow rates they are probably also able to deliver some positive end expiratory pressure (PEEP), which can be advantageous for hypoxic children (e.g. pneumonia, pulmonary contusion, and bronchiolitis).

Methods of assisted ventilation

If a child stops breathing completely or if spontaneous ventilation is inadequate, positive pressure ventilation support is required.

When providing positive pressure ventilation for an infant/child, aim for a respiratory rate of 12–20 min^{-1} with younger children having higher rates (except during cardiorespiratory arrest when ventilation rates of 10–12 min^{-1} should be delivered to infants and children). In a newborn the rate should be 30 min^{-1}. The volume delivered should be sufficient to produce a normal visible chest expansion and breath sounds on auscultation. Continuous monitoring of the heart rate and SpO$_2$ should be undertaken as soon as practicable.

Mouth-to-mask devices

Rescuers should not delay giving rescue breaths until the arrival of advanced paediatric airway and ventilation equipment, and therefore expired air breaths (e.g. mouth-to-mouth) using a barrier device such as a face shield may be more appropriate in initial resuscitation attempts. The pocket mask is widely used in resuscitation of apnoeic adults and the standard size may be suitable for use in larger children and adolescents. There is a 'paediatric' pocket mask available but "one size" does not fit all infants and children, and an appropriate size of paediatric facemask may need to be substituted. Expired air ventilation using a pocket mask should only be used if a manual ventilation device (e.g. self-inflating bag system) is not immediately available.

When it is deemed appropriate for use (e.g. in an adolescent) the pocket mask is a device designed to minimise infection risks when delivering expired air ventilation. The device is made of transparent plastic with a one-way valve that directs the patient's expired breath away from the rescuer. An oxygen delivery port (which also has a one-way valve) is incorporated into some pocket masks and allows supplemental oxygen to be administered.

Technique for mouth-to-mask ventilation:

- Having assembled the pocket mask, the rescuer positions themselves behind the supine child.

- The child's head should be placed in an appropriate position (e.g. 'sniffing' position) to achieve a patent airway.

- Apply the mask over the child's mouth and nose, pressing down with the thumbs of both hands to create a seal.

- Lift the child's jaw upwards (jaw thrust) into the mask with the other fingers, taking care not to compress the soft tissues under the mandible.

- Blow through the mask's one-way valve until chest expansion is observed (Figure 4.10).

- Stop inflation and observe the chest falling.

- Repeat as appropriate.

- If chest expansion is not seen, assess whether this may be due to inadequate airway patency or a poor seal between the child's face and the mask, and correct as necessary.

- If the mask has an appropriate port and there is oxygen available, supplemental oxygen should be administered.

This technique can also be used with a standard facemask, but it will not provide protection against infection unless a breathing system filter is also used.

The self-inflating bag device (as used for bag-mask ventilation)

In a child who has inadequate/absent breathing, maintenance of a patent airway is the first priority of management. Once this is achieved, adequate ventilation

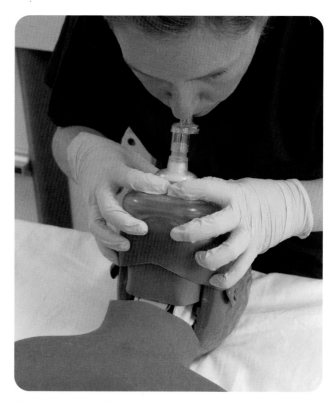

Figure 4.10 Ventilation with a pocket mask

must be established. The self-inflating bag system with an oxygen reservoir is the first line system for providing ventilation during resuscitation. Although the self-inflating bag can be used without a supplemental oxygen source, in resuscitation situations it is usually used to deliver ventilation with high flow oxygen. The self-inflating bag can be connected not only to a facemask but also to a tracheal tube or laryngeal mask airway when these are in place.

The self-inflating bag operates in the following manner:

Inspiration – squeezing of the bag allows oxygen enriched air to flow through a one way inspiratory (non-rebreathing) valve at the patient end of the device and hence to the patient. A valve at the oxygen port/reservoir end of the system prevents gases entering the reservoir bag.

Expiration – when the squeezing pressure on the bag is stopped, passively expired gases from the patient pass out into the atmosphere through the non-rebreathing valve at the patient end of the device. The bag reinflates, owing to its elastic recoil, and oxygen enters the bag via the oxygen port and via the reservoir bag so increasing the oxygen concentration in the bag.

Used without supplemental oxygen, a self-inflating bag system will ventilate with room air (21% oxygen). The oxygen concentration can be increased to approximately 50% by attaching a high flow of oxygen to the oxygen port on the base of the bag, without a reservoir bag. The use of the reservoir bag, as described above together with high-flow of oxygen at 15 L min^{-1}, will enable the delivery of > 90% oxygen (Figure 4.11).

Self-inflating bags are available in four sizes (generally 250, 450–500, 900–1200 and 1600–2000 mL). The two smallest sizes usually have a pressure-limiting valve that prevents excessive inflation pressures that otherwise may cause barotrauma. The pressure limit is pre-determined by the manufacturers (usually 30–40 cm H_2O). During resuscitation, higher than normal inflation pressures may be required and the pressure limiting valve may need to be over-ridden. The most common reason for needing to activate the pressure-limiting valve is upper airway obstruction due to a poor airway opening technique. Thus ensure that the child's airway is patent (e.g. check head positioning) before overriding the valve. It should be noted that such valves are now being incorporated into some of the large bag sizes.

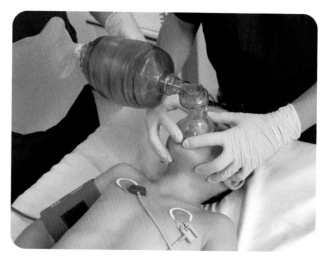

Figure 4.11 Ventilation of a child with a self-inflating bag-mask device

The smallest bag (250 mL) is intended for use in preterm neonates < 2.5 kg only. It is not appropriate for use in full term neonates and infants as it may be inadequate to support effective tidal volume.

The second size of bag (450–500 mL) is generally most appropriate for full term neonates, infants and pre-schoolchildren. Many paediatric hospitals will also stock the 900–1200 mL size bags for school age children/early adolescence as the largest size (1600–2000 mL) can be more unwieldy to use. Regardless of size the provider should only use the force and tidal volume necessary to cause visible chest expansion (Figures 4.11, 4.12).

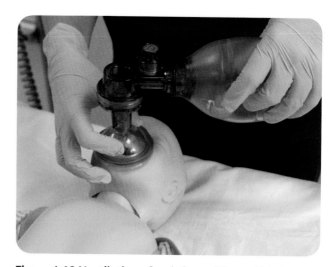

Figure 4.12 Ventilation of an infant with a self-inflating bag-mask device

Self-inflating bags should not be used to deliver oxygen to spontaneously breathing patients. Depending on the valve system, this may result in the inspiration of room air (or even rebreathing of the child's own passively expired air if the mask is held tightly on the face) as the child's own respiratory efforts may not generate sufficient pressure to open the valve. Children, who are making adequate respiratory effort, should therefore have oxygen administered by another method.

Facemask selection

These are the interface between the ventilation device and the child. They must be capable of providing a good seal over the mouth and nose whilst ensuring minimal pressure is applied over the eyes.

Masks are available in a variety of sizes and two basic types; anatomically shaped ones for older children and adults, and circular ones for infants and small children (Figure 4.13). The preferred mask is transparent (to allow rapid detection of secretions/vomit and observation of the child's central colour) and should have a low dead space.

Bag-mask ventilation

Ventilatory support using assisted ventilation is indicated in the child with decompensated respiratory failure. Bag-mask ventilation (BMV) describes the use of a facemask and a self-inflating bag system with an oxygen reservoir attached that delivers positive pressure ventilation without rebreathing of expired respiratory gases, as described above.

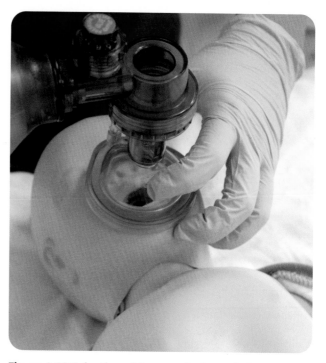

Figure 4.13 Selection of face masks for an infant

Correctly performed BMV is an important skill for all healthcare professionals who work with children. Whilst the operating principle of self-inflating bags is simple, they require skill and practice to use them safely and effectively.

Hypoventilation can occur with poor technique (e.g. inadequate mask seal or incorrect head positioning) and is likely to have a negative effect on outcome.

Excessive BMV should be avoided as it causes over insufflation of the stomach. Gastric distension will then limit the movement of the diaphragm and therefore reduce ventilation. It will also lead to an increased risk of gastro-oesophageal reflux and aspiration of gastric contents.

When self-inflating bags are used with a facemask, it can be difficult for a single rescuer to achieve an airtight seal whilst simultaneously using one hand to maintain a patent airway with a jaw thrust manoeuvre, and squeezing the bag with the other. A two-person technique (one person to maintain the airway and hold the mask in position, and the second to squeeze the bag) will usually overcome these difficulties The effectiveness of BMV can be seen by observing adequate chest expansion, monitoring heart rate, auscultation of the chest and SpO_2 monitoring.

Technique for bag-mask ventilation

- Having selected the appropriate size of bag and mask, the rescuer should stand behind the supine child.

- The oxygen supply should be connected at a high flow and the reservoir bag should be seen to inflate.

- If there is a second person available they should stand at one side of the child.

- The child's head should be placed in an appropriate position (e.g. 'neutral' position for an infant, 'sniffing the morning air' in the older child) to achieve a patent airway. A roll placed under the infant's shoulders is often useful to assist in maintaining an appropriate airway position (unless contraindicated in trauma cases).

- Apply the mask over the child's mouth and nose, gently pressing down with the thumb and index finger of one hand (or both hands if two rescuers).

- Lift the child's jaw upwards (jaw thrust) into the mask with the other fingers, with one finger under the angle of the jaw. Take care not to compress the soft tissues underneath the mandible.

- Gently squeeze the bag until chest expansion is observed to a normal chest expansion.

- Stop inflation and observe the chest falling.

- Repeat as appropriate.

- If chest expansion is not seen, assess whether this may be due to inadequate airway patency or a poor seal

between the child's face and the mask, and correct as necessary.

Bag-mask ventilation frequently results in gastric distension, and therefore placement of a gastric tube should be undertaken as early as practicable.

T-piece (flow-inflating bag) circuit

This equipment is often employed by anaesthesia and critical care staff. It requires a continuous gas source for inflation of the bag, and therefore there must always be an appropriate self-inflating system immediately available, in case there is a failure of the gas supply. This circuit does not have any valves and the bag has an open end. To achieve ventilation the end of the bag needs to be occluded and the bag squeezed. To prevent rebreathing a high gas flow is required (at least three times the minute ventilation of the patient (i.e. > 30 mL kg^{-1} x respiratory rate). This circuit can deliver 100% oxygen and can be used in spontaneously breathing children. The bag of this device gives some 'feeling' of the compliance of the lungs and allows some positive end expiratory pressure (PEEP) to be applied manually. The safe and effective use of this equipment requires considerable expertise and it should be utilised by experienced practitioners only.

Supraglottic upper airway devices:

Laryngeal mask airway (LMA)

The LMA is a supraglottic airway device, which is widely used in children undergoing routine surgical procedures as a means of providing an effective airway to achieve ventilation and oxygenation (Figure 4.14). Like the oropharyngeal airway, it can cause gagging, coughing and laryngospasm in children who are semi-conscious, so it should only be used in unconscious patients with relaxed jaw muscles.

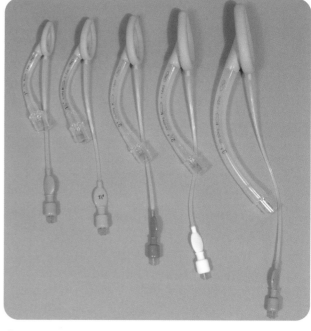

Figure 4.14 Laryngeal mask airways

Trained providers should consider LMA insertion if BMV is difficult or not successful. It is an alternative to tracheal intubation when suitably skilled individuals are not available.

It consists of a tube with an inflatable cuffed mask at the distal end, which is introduced into the mouth and advanced into the pharynx, until resistance is felt (Figure 4.15). The cuff is then inflated, providing a low pressure seal over the laryngeal inlet. This leaves the distal opening of the tube just above the vocal cords. The LMA does not protect the lungs from regurgitation and aspiration of gastric contents.

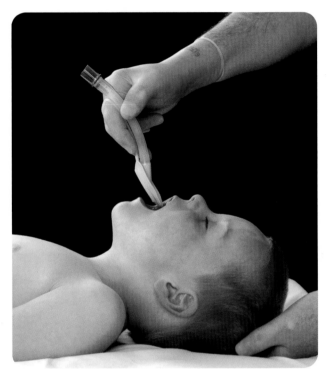

Figure 4.15 Insertion of laryngeal mask airway

LMA insertion technique

The correct size of LMA is based on the age/weight of the child (Table 4.2). Prior to insertion the device should be inspected for damage and tubing obstruction. The cuff should be checked for leaks by inflation to 50% greater than the recommended inflation volume. A water soluble lubricant gel needs to be applied to the tip and back of the cuff, just before insertion.

There have been several methods described to insert the LMA in children. In general it is useful to consider the LMA as slightly longer oropharyngeal airway with the distal cuff sitting over the laryngeal inlet.

The following is the standard insertion technique:

- The cuff is fully deflated and the tubing is held by the dominant hand of the rescuer, just above the cuff (Figure 4.15).

- Whilst standing behind the child's head, the other hand holds the occiput and gently extends the head.

- The tip of the mask is inserted into the child's mouth and is pressed against the hard palate.

- The mask is advanced into the mouth until the cuff passes beyond the back of the tongue. Stop pushing the mask once resistance is felt (the cuff should not be visible in the mouth once the mask is in place).

- Once the LMA is correctly positioned, the cuff should be slowly inflated using an air filled syringe (Table 4.2).

- A small outward movement of the tube is frequently seen once the correct volume is given, this is the moment to stop inflating the cuff.

- The opening of the cuff must be facing forward once the LMA is inserted to lie above the laryngeal inlet (i.e. towards the patient's feet).

- A self-inflating bag system is connected to the LMA and gentle squeezed. The chest should be seen to rise in a similar manner to that when performing BMV.

- The LMA should be secured in place using tape.

If resistance is felt while attempting to pass the cuff beyond the back of the tongue, various strategies can be used to aid insertion. The head can be further extended, the mask partially inflated and rotated 90° or 180° (like the rotation technique used to insert an oropharyngeal airway) and then further advanced. If the chest is not seen to rise the LMA should be removed and BMV should be performed.

Table 4.2 LMA size selection and cuff volume		
LMA Size	**Child selection**	**Maximum cuff volume**
1	Neonates < 5 kg	4 mL
1 ½	Infants 5–10 kg	7 mL
2	Infants 10–20 kg	10 mL
2 ½	Children 20–30 kg	14 mL
3	Children 30–50 kg	20 mL

Other supraglottic airway devices

There are now several other SGAs (e.g. i-gel, LMA-supreme), which have been used successfully in children under anaesthesia. They may also be useful in resuscitation. Providers should use the equipment they are familiar with.

Tracheal intubation

Tracheal intubation should only be performed by experienced personnel who have been trained to perform the technique. It is considered the "gold standard" method to achieve and maintain a secure airway. In addition, it allows optimal control of the ventilation pressures (including PEEP), prevents gastric distension, protects the lungs from aspiration of gastric contents, and makes it easier to ventilate the lungs when chest compressions are performed. The oral route is quicker and simpler than nasal intubation, whereas the nasal route provides a more secure airway.

Tracheal intubation should be considered in the following situations:

- Ineffective BMV
- Severe anatomical or functional upper airways obstruction (e.g. facial burns)
- Need for protection of the airway from aspiration of gastric contents
- If high pressures are required to maintain adequate oxygenation (e.g. asthma)
- Mechanical ventilation is required
- Need for bronchial or tracheal suctioning
- Instability or high probability of one of the above occurring before or during transport

Intubation can be more difficult in children compared to intubating adults. It requires extensive training, both on manikins and on real patients in the operating theatre or intensive care unit. In most situations, provided there is effective ventilation using BMV, there is no need to perform tracheal intubation until experienced personnel are available. In some circumstances (e.g. head trauma and cervical spine injury), repeated attempts at intubation by the inexperienced may worsen the child's condition.

Equipment

Tracheal tubes

Traditionally uncuffed tubes have been preferred for intubation for children up to eight years (up to 6 mm internal diameter). In these children the cricoid ring is the narrowest part of the airway and acts as a 'natural cuff'. However, recent studies have shown that there is no greater risk of complications for children between one month and eight years when cuffed tracheal tubes (TT) are used. Consequently cuffed TT can be considered for use in resuscitation of infants and children (except neonates) provided the correct tube size is selected, the cuff inflation pressure is monitored (20–25 cm H_2O) and the tube position verified. If a cuffed TT is used, the cuff should be of a high volume, low-pressure design and should be positioned below the cricoid ring, with the tracheal tube tip above the carina. Under certain circumstances (e.g. poor lung compliance, high airway resistance or a large glottic air leak) cuffed TT have distinct advantages over uncuffed tubes.

Regardless of whether a cuffed or uncuffed TT is used, its position should be checked to ensure that the tip of the tube lies above the carina. Tracheal tubes have markings along their length that indicate the distance the tube needs to pass, along the larynx of an average child, to rest in mid-trachea.

Choice of tracheal tube

Tube sizes are based on internal diameter (ID) in millimetres:

- preterm neonates: 2.5–3.0 mm (or gestational weeks/10)
- term neonates: 3.0–3.5 mm
- infants < one year: 4.0–4.5 mm.

Children over one year: appropriate ID is given by the formula for uncuffed TT:

$$\frac{\text{Age (years)}}{4} + 4$$

Ensure a half size larger and smaller TT are available to hand.

If a cuffed TT is used, a half size smaller diameter should be used.

Resuscitation tapes (e.g. Broselow, Sandell tapes) can also be used to estimate the TT size based on the child's length.

To estimate the length of TT for correct placement in the trachea, the following formulae can be used:

$$\text{Oral TT: length (cm)} = \frac{\text{Age (years)}}{2} + 12$$

or, up to 12 years, 3 x ID (cm).

$$\text{Nasal TT: length (cm)} = \frac{\text{Age (years)}}{2} + 15$$

Clinical and radiological confirmation of tube placement is essential following intubation.

Stylet

A stylet moulds the shape of TT during intubation to facilitate its direction into the glottis. It must be chosen according to TT size and should be fixed so that its tip does not protrude beyond the distal end of the tube (to avoid tracheal trauma).

Laryngoscope

This consists of a body containing batteries, a light source and a blade. It must be checked prior to use and spares must always be available.

There are two types of blades; curved and straight (Figure 4.16). Their role is the same, that is, to keep the tongue out of the way and to displace the epiglottis so allowing the vocal cords to be seen.

The choice of blade type depends on personal preference and the experience of the provider, but the following age limits can act as a guide.

Straight blades (numbers 0 and 1) are usually preferred for infants (< one year) and neonates, and are designed to lift the epiglottis under the tip of the blade so that the vocal cords can be seen. The blade may also be placed in the vallecula (between the tongue base and the epiglottis). The advantage of lifting the epiglottis is that it will then not obscure the view of the vocal cords.

Curved blades are preferred in children and adolescents (numbers 0, 1 and 2 for infants and children; 3 and 4 for adolescents and adults). They are designed to have their tip resting in the vallecula and to lift the epiglottis from above.

Straight and curved blades come in several lengths. The choice of length is guided by the child's age. If in doubt, remember that it is possible to intubate with a blade that is too long but not with one that is too short.

Videolaryngoscopes are becoming widely available and are especially useful in the management of the difficult airway (e.g. congenital airway problems, trauma, burns).

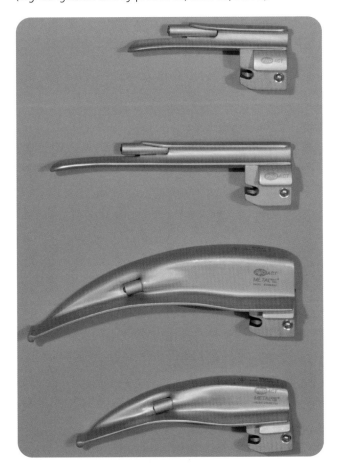

Figure 4.16 Larnygoscope blades

Procedure

The ECG, heart rate and SpO_2 should be monitored during intubation. There is a risk of reflex bradycardia and hypoxia during intubation. Peripheral oxygen saturation is unreliable if peripheral perfusion is inadequate (e.g. in cardiorespiratory arrest, shock or circulatory failure).

Check all necessary equipment is available before intubation:

- medications

- self-inflating bag system and oxygen supply

- oropharyngeal/nasopharyngeal airway

- laryngoscope handles and blades

- tracheal tubes of the appropriate sizes

- end-tidal CO_2 monitoring

- stylet and Magill forceps

- suction apparatus with appropriate size of suckers

- tapes or ties to secure the tube

- nasogastric tubes.

Intubation technique

Prior to intubation, the patient should be ventilated with 100% oxygen by BMV. If during the intubation attempt there is either a fall in peripheral oxygen saturation or bradycardia occurs, the procedure should be interrupted and the patient ventilated again with 100% oxygen by BMV.

In cardiorespiratory arrest, intubation should be performed as soon as the equipment and experienced personnel are available.

In infants < one year, head and neck extension may be required by placing a neck roll under the shoulders (provided there is no history of cervical spine injury).

If there is suspected cervical spine injury, in-line manual immobilisation of the neck should be maintained at all times during intubation.

Attempts to intubate should be interrupted if:

- the peripheral oxygen saturations reading begins to fall

- the heart rate begins to fall or is < 60 min^{-1}

- more than 30 s has elapsed

BMV should be recommenced until the child's condition improves before attempting intubation again.

An incorrectly placed tube or prolonged hypoxia from repeated intubation attempts can cause morbidity and even mortality.

Verification of TT placement

Displaced, misplaced or obstructed TT occur frequently and can lead to an increased risk of death. The position of the tube should be checked after placement using end-tidal CO_2 monitoring (e.g. capnography). CO_2 should be detected if the TT is correctly placed after four to six ventilations. If after these ventilations no end-tidal carbon dioxide is present then the TT is likely to be in the oesophagus and not in the trachea. The tube should be immediately removed and BMV restarted, as the patient is at risk of hypoxia.

Confirmation of correct TT placement comprises:

- clear visualisation of tube passing through glottis
- end-tidal carbon dioxide monitoring
- symmetrical chest rise and fall with each ventilation
- bilateral air entry in four zones with each ventilation – axillae and apices
- absence of bubbling noise over the stomach upon ventilation
- chest X-ray (after initial resuscitation) to confirm TT is above the carina (ideally tip between T2 and T3).

Once the correct position is confirmed, secure the TT with tape after drying and cleaning the skin with gauze.

If auscultation is asymmetrical, and particularly if it is decreased on the left side of the chest, withdraw the TT cautiously by 0.5 cm increments until symmetrical breath sounds are heard. If breath sounds are now heard bilaterally, then the TT will have been in the right main bronchus before adjustment.

Sudden deterioration of the intubated patient

If the condition of an intubated child deteriorates, consider various possibilities, which are easily recalled by the acronym 'DOPES':

D displacement of the TT (accidental extubation or TT in the right main bronchus)

O obstruction of the TT (secretions or kinking), filter or tubing

P pneumothorax and other pulmonary disorders (bronchospasm, oedema, pulmonary hypertension)

E equipment failure (check source of oxygen, ventilation bag, ventilator etc.)

S stomach (distension can alter diaphragm mechanics)

Other reasons for deterioration or inadequate ventilation include:

- TT too small with significant air leak
- tidal volume given too small
- pressure-limiting valve active with non-compliant lungs (e.g. in near drowning).

Emergency anaesthesia for intubation

In cardiorespiratory arrest, as the child is unconscious, intubation does not require analgesia, anaesthesia or neuromuscular blockade (muscle relaxants). In many other emergency situations, however, combinations of these drugs may be required.

Emergency anaesthesia is delivered by a combination of drugs to facilitate and secure tracheal intubation in an emergency. It reduces the incidence of adverse events in responsive patients. These include:

- hypoxia
- pain
- cardiac arrhythmias
- rise in systemic BP and intracranial pressure
- airway trauma
- reflux and aspiration of gastric contents
- psychological trauma.

Pre-oxygenation is important to prevent hypoxia during emergency anaesthesia and intubation, with at least three minutes of oxygen delivered by BMV or an anaesthetic circuit to increase the amount of oxygen reserve. A checklist should be used and the team briefed before embarking on the procedure to minimise complications. Emergency drugs, including atropine, should be immediately available. A combination of drugs in table 4.3 should then be administered by the team.

The team delivering emergency anaesthesia must have considerable experience in intubation and BMV, as the child will not be able to breathe on their own after the drugs have been administered. An alternative plan for airway management in case of unsuccessful intubation must have been considered during the checklist and brief.

Table 4.3 Some examples of drugs for emergency anaesthesia		
Analgesia	**Anaesthetic agent**	**Neuromusclar blocking drug**
Alfentanil Fentanyl	Thiopentone Ketamine Propofol Sevoflurane	Suxamethonium Rocuronium

Care of the child with a tracheostomy

A tracheostomy is a surgical opening into the trachea, which bypasses the mouth, pharynx and larynx. Children may have a tracheostomy present because of a congenital upper airway narrowing or to facilitate long-term ventilation. They often have complex medical problems and information about this should be gained as soon as possible. The parents/caregivers will have been taught how to care for the tracheostomy, including emergencies, and paediatric basic life support.

The ABCDE method should be used when assessing children with a tracheostomy and resuscitation should be started as usual if no breathing and/or pulse are detected. The main differences to the management of the airway/breathing are discussed below.

In these children, difficulty in breathing leading to respiratory distress may be caused by obstruction of the tracheostomy tube leading to ineffective ventilation. The management of an obstructed tracheostomy is detailed in Figure 4.17. Try to relieve the obstruction by suctioning the tracheostomy tube. If this is unsuccessful, the tracheostomy tube should be removed immediately and replaced; if a clean tube is not available, ventilation via BMV should be given at the tracheostomy stoma site until the tube is cleaned and replaced. If the child's upper airway is patent, it may be possible to provide bag-mask ventilation via the mouth and nose using a conventional bag and mask whilst the tracheal stoma site is occluded. In an emergency situation, tracheal intubation via the tracheostomy with a classical endotracheal tube may be needed. Attention should be given to correct positioning (not endobronchial).

Cricoid pressure (Sellick manoeuvre)

Unconscious children with a full stomach are at risk of regurgitation of gastric contents and pulmonary aspiration. The application of pressure to the cricoid cartilage occludes the oesophagus, reducing the risk of regurgitation and can be used during BMV and attempts at intubation. Cricoid pressure is difficult to perform correctly in infants and young children however, and may cause airway distortion and obstruction. If it is thought the airway is in any way compromised, cricoid pressure should be removed immediately.

Cricoid pressure is performed by:

- identification of the cricoid cartilage (just below the thyroid cartilage)

- gentle application of pressure using two fingers to the cricoid cartilage

- the cricoid is displaced backwards to compress the oesophagus

N.B. This manoeuvre should not be performed if the child begins actively to vomit because it may lead to oesophageal rupture.

The difficult airway

If ventilation is not possible using BMV, call for assistance and perform simple airway manoeuvres. In the majority of situations it should be possible to ventilate the child until expert assistance arrives.

Occasionally, despite using these simple airway manoeuvres, ventilation may not be possible due to airway abnormalities (e.g. facial trauma, epiglottitis, airway malformations).

If the obstruction is above the larynx (facial trauma, congenital facial abnormalities), supra-glottic airway devices (e.g. LMA) can be lifesaving.

Nevertheless, expert help should be sought immediately as intubation may be needed using either conventional or optical laryngoscopy. Intubation by the non-expert would only be acceptable if no such expertise were available and it is not otherwise possible to oxygenate and ventilate a hypoxic child.

In the very rare situations when the clinician cannot ventilate the child and intubation is not possible, cricothyroidotomy should be considered.

Cricothyroidotomy

Needle cricothyroidotomy is a 'last resort' emergency technique indicated in cases of upper airway obstruction (e.g. laryngeal obstruction by oedema, foreign body or major facial trauma) and is a technique of default (i.e. only to be undertaken when ventilation by BMV or LMA and TT intubation have failed).

Cricothyroidotomy can be performed with a large-bore over-the-needle cannula. A syringe is connected to the cannula and gently aspirated as it punctures either a prominent tracheal ring or the cricothyroid membrane percutaneously, at an angle of 45° from the head; these landmarks can be very difficult to identify in pre-school children. The trachea is situated just beneath the skin. Air aspiration confirms the correct position. The needle is removed and the cannula connected to a 3 or 3.5 mm TT adaptator and thence to a self-inflating bag system. An alternative is to connect directly via a 3-way tap, with all ports open to an oxygen source. Oxygen is given by obstructing the side port of the 3-way tap for 1 s and allowing 4 s for exhalation.

Oxygen flow for this technique in L min^{-1} = age of the child in years (maximum 6 L min^{-1}).

Over-the-needle cannulae have high resistances. Small tidal volumes are delivered and there is no significant CO_2 removal. There is also a risk of barotrauma, particularly so with the 3-way tap technique, if the airway is completely obstructed above the cannula. The technique only provides temporary oxygenation until a definitive airway can be provided. Expert help must be sought as soon as possible.

Surgical tracheostomy should be reserved for skilled practitioners because it is a difficult technique with major risks, including haemorrhage, laryngeal tear, pneumomediastinum and subcutaneous emphysema.

Emergency Paediatric Tracheostomy Management

Basic Response

SAFETY – STIMULATE – SHOUT FOR HELP – OXYGEN

SAFE: Check Safe area, Stimulate, and Shout for help, CALL 2222 (hospital) or 999 (home)
AIRWAY: Open child's airway: head tilt / chin lift / pillow or towel under shoulders may help
OXYGEN: Ensure high flow oxygen to the tracheostomy AND the face as soon as oxygen available
Capnograph: Exhaled carbon dioxide waveform may indicate a patent airway (secondary responders)

SUCTION TO ASSESS TRACHEOSTOMY PATENCY

Remove any attachments: humidifier (HME), speaking valve and change inner tube (if present)
Inner tubes need re-inserting to connect to bagging circuits

Can you pass a SUCTION catheter? **YES**

The tracheostomy tube is patent
Perform tracheal suction
Consider partial obstruction
Consider tracheostomy tube change
CONTINUE ASSESSMENT (ABCDE)

NO

EMERGENCY TRACHEOSTOMY TUBE CHANGE

Deflate cuff (if present). Reassess patency after any tube change
1st – same size tube, 2nd – smaller size tube
*3rd – smaller size tube sited over suction catheter to guide
IF UNSUCCESSFUL – REMOVE THE TUBE

IS THE PATIENT BREATHING? Look, listen and feel at the mouth and tracheostomy/stoma

NO **YES**

5 RESCUE BREATHS – USE TRACHEOSTOMY IF PATENT

Patent Upper Airway – deliver breath to the mouth
Obstructed Upper Airway – deliver breath to tracheostomy/stoma

RESPONDS:
Continue oxygen, reassessment and stabilisation

NO

CHECK FOR SIGNS OF LIFE ? – START CPR

15 compressions: 2 rescue breaths
Ensure help or resuscitation team called

Plan for definitive airway if tube change failure

Advanced Response

Primary emergency oxygenation

Standard **ORAL airway** manoeuvres **may be appropriate.**
If so **cover the stoma** (swabs/hand).
Use: Bag-valve-face mask
   Oral or nasal airway adjuncts
   Supraglottic airway device
   e.g. Laryngeal Mask Airway (LMA)

Tracheostomy STOMA ventilation
   Paediatric face mask applied to stoma
   LMA applied to stoma

Secondary emergency oxygenation

ORAL intubation may be appropriate with a downsized ET tube
Uncut tube, advanced beyond stoma
Prepare for difficult intubation
'Difficult Airway' Expert and Equipment

Attempt intubation of STOMA
3.0 ID tracheostomy tube/ETT
'Difficult Airway' Expert and Equipment

****EQUIPMENT: Fibreoptic scope, bougie, airway exchange catheter, Airway trolley**

*3-smaller size tube sited over suction catheter to guide: to be used if out of hospital

Figure 4.17 Emergency Paediatric Tracheostomy Management – resuscitation algorithm for a patient with a tracheostomy; NTSP Paediatric Working Group, Sep 2014

Pulse oximetry

The clinical recognition of cyanosis may be difficult and is not reliable. Pulse oximetry enables continuous evaluation of the peripheral oxygen saturation of haemoglobin and is a valuable non-invasive method of monitoring the child (Chapter 2). It provides an early indication of hypoxia and should be used during both stabilisation and transportation of the critically ill child (Figure 4.18). A detecting probe is placed around a finger/toe (in the child) or hand/foot (in the infant). Ideally the pulse oximeter monitor should display a wave-form, a numerical percentage of oxygenation and produce a tone modulated sound. It is important to remember that it is a measure of oxygenation and does not indicate the adequacy of ventilation. Peripheral oxygen saturation readings should always be interpreted with reference to the inspired oxygen concentration. When peripheral perfusion is poor, recorded values will be unreliable. Furthermore in situations of cardiorespiratory arrest, circulatory failure or shock with severely reduced peripheral perfusion, pulse oximetry may be unrecordable.

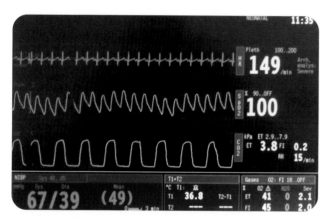

Figure 4.18 Pulse oximetry and capnography

End-tidal carbon dioxide monitoring (capnography)

Monitoring end-tidal CO_2 reliably confirms TT placement in a child weighing more than 2 kg with a perfusing rhythm. It should be used following intubation and during the transportation of an intubated child. It can also be used in non-intubated critically ill children (e.g. non-invasive ventilation, nasal cannulae). The presence of an end-tidal CO_2 trace after 4–6 ventilated breaths indicates that the TT is in the tracheobronchial tree, both in the presence of a perfusing rhythm and during cardiorespiratory arrest. Figure 4.18 shows an example of an end-tidal CO_2 trace.

The absence of exhaled CO_2 during cardiorespiratory arrest however, does not prove that the TT is misplaced, as pulmonary blood flow may be very low. If exhaled CO_2 is not detected during CPR, the TT position should be confirmed using other methods (e.g. direct visualisation, bilateral air entry); if TT position is confirmed and correct then CPR quality may be inadequate. If there is doubt

though, the TT should be removed and BMV used to ventilate the patient instead.

Types of end-tidal carbon dioxide sampling devices

1. Side-stream end-tidal CO_2

A connector is placed in the breathing system, usually at the end of the tracheal tube or supraglottic airway – the closer to the airway device the better. A fine bore sampling tube then takes a continuous sample and analyses it with infrared light. The amount of infrared light absorbed is proportional to the amount of CO_2 present. This is then presented as a number (capnometry) or graphically (capnography). The latter gives more clinical information.

2. Main-stream end-tidal CO_2

The infrared source and detector are contained within a cell or cuvette which is placed directly in the breathing system, usually between the TT or SGA and the ventilation tubing. Gas is analysed as it passes through the sensor and none is removed from the system (unlike side stream). This usually presents the information as capnography. The disadvantage of this type of device is its size and weight, especially in small children – there is a risk of TT dislodgement.

Information that can be gained from end-tidal CO_2 monitoring during resuscitation

1. Tube placement – this is the most reliable method to confirm correct TT placement.

2. Quality of CPR – the more effective chest compressions are the greater the cardiac output which delivers CO_2 to the lungs where it is exhaled thus generating a higher end-tidal concentration.

3. Return of spontaneous circulation (ROSC) – there will be an immediate sustained increase in end-tidal CO_2. This may be the first indicator of ROSC and often precedes a palpable pulse.

4. Guide to the rate of ventilation – hyperventilation is common during resuscitation and should be avoided. End-tidal CO_2 can help avoid this.

Eich C, Roessler M, Nemeth M, Russo SG, Heuer JF, Timmermann A. Characteristics and outcome of prehospital paediatric tracheal intubation attended by anaesthesia-trained emergency physicians. Resuscitation 2009;80:1371-7.

Ghai B, Wig J. Comparison of different techniques of laryngeal mask placement in children. Curr opin Anesth 2009; 22:4000-404.

Grein AJ, Weiner GM. Laryngeal mask airway versus bag-mask ventilation or endotracheal intubation for neonatal resuscitation. Cochrane Database Systemic Review 2005; CD003314.
http://www2.cochrane.org/reviews/en/ab003314

Warner KJ, et al. Prehospital management of the difficult airway: a prospective cohort study. J Emerg Med 2009;36:257-65.

Weiss M, Dullenkopf A, Fischer JE, Keller C, Gerber AC European Paediatric Endotracheal Intubation Study Group. Prospective randomized controlled multi-centre trial of cuffed or uncuffed endotracheal tubes in small children. Br J Anaesth. 2009;103:867-73.

Zelicof-Paul A, Smith-Lockridge A, Schnadower D et al. Controversies in rapid sequence intubation in children. Current Opinion in Pediatrics 2005;17: 355-362.

Summary learning

- **Airway management is the first priority in the care of the critically ill or injured child and is central to successful paediatric resuscitation.**
- **The delivery of high flow oxygen with the use of simple airway manoeuvres and BMV provides effective first-line management in the critically ill child.**
- **Tracheal intubation is reserved for those experienced in the technique because it has many complications.**

My key take-home messages from this chapter

Further reading

Blevin AE, McDouall SF, Rechner JA, Saunders TA, Barber VS, Young JD, Mason DG.A comparison of the laryngeal mask airway with the facemask and oropharyngeal airway for manual ventilation by first responders in children. Anaesthesia. 2009;64:1312-6.

Bhende MS, Thompson AE. Evaluation of an endtidal carbon dioxide detector during pediatric cardiopulmonary resuscitation. Pediatrics 1995; 95:395-399.

De Caen AR, Kleinman ME et al. Part 10: Pediatric basic and advanced life support 2010 International Consensus on Cardiopulmonary Rescucitation and Cardiovascular Care Science with Treatment Recommendations. Resuscitation 2010;81s:e213-259.

Ellis DY, et al. Cricoid pressure in emergency department rapid sequence tracheal intubations: a risk-benefit analysis. Ann Emerg Med 2007;50:653-65.

Gausche M, Lewis RJ, Stratton SJ, et al. Effect of out-of-hospital pediatric endotracheal intubation on survival and neurological outcome: a controlled clinical trial. JAMA 2000;283:783-90.

Advanced management of circulation and drugs

Contents

- **Establishment of circulatory access**
- **Fluid administration**
- **First-line resuscitation medications**

Learning outcomes

To enable you to:

- **Consider the requirement for circulatory access during resuscitation**
- **Describe the different routes of emergency circulatory access and their appropriate use**
- **Discuss the advantages and potential complications of intraosseous access**
- **Understand the type and volume of fluids to be administered in the emergency situation**
- **Understand the indications, dosages and actions of the first-line medications used in cardiorespiratory arrest**

Circulatory access

Once the airway is patent and adequate ventilation of the child is established, attention must be focused on circulation. The exception to this is for the child who presents with life-threatening haemorrhage when circulation would be attended to simultaneously with A and B assessment by a trauma team.

Establish circulatory access within the first few minutes of resuscitation or following the recognition of signs of shock in order that:

- medications can be given (e.g. adrenaline)

- fluids can be given

- blood samples can be obtained.

Circulatory access may be achieved via the intravenous (IV) or intraosseous (IO) routes. In cardiorespiratory arrest and/or severe shock states when peripheral circulation is severely compromised the IO route is the preferred method of gaining vascular access. The tracheal route is no longer recommended because of the variability in alveolar drug absorption.

For children who are unwell but remain responsive to pain, IV access is preferred over IO if possible, as infusions of fluids and drugs via the IO route can be painful. If there is an IV cannula already in situ, check its patency before use otherwise insert the largest possible IV cannula in peripheral veins (e.g. the antecubital fossa, the long saphenous vein or the back of the hand (or feet in smaller children)).

EPALS

The use of scalp veins during resuscitation is not advisable due to the risk of extravasation leading to potential tissue necrosis. Their use may also interfere with the management of the airway and ventilation. If the child requires chest compressions these should not be interrupted by access attempts or other procedures apart from defibrillation.

Catecholamines (e.g. adrenaline, noradrenaline, dopamine) should ideally be infused through a dedicated line; continuous catecholamine therapy may be required as part of the ongoing resuscitation of the child.

Intraosseous access

IO access is indicated in children, infants, or newborns in any clinical situation where vascular access is urgently required but not immediately available via a peripheral vein. This may include cardiorespiratory arrest, shock, life-threatening status epilepticus, burns and oedema.

In these situations gaining vascular access via the IO route rather than the peripheral, umbilical or central routes may be safer, faster to achieve and associated with fewer complications. It requires less skill and practice on the part of practitioners who may use the techniques only rarely.

Often IV access is easier to obtain once a fluid bolus and medications have been administered via the IO needle. Although IO needles can remain in place for up to 72 h they are usually removed as soon as another means of vascular access (either peripheral or central) is available.

IO needles are usually placed in the proximal or distal ends of long bones . The IO needle is inserted through the skin, periosteum, then cortex of the bone so that the needle lies in the medullary (or marrow) cavity. The medullary cavity provides access to a non-collapsible venous plexus which drains into the central venous circulation. When accessed with an IO needle, medications and fluid will pass from the medullary space through the vascular system into the central circulation (Figure 5.1).

The main advantages of IO access are:

- The relative ease and speed of insertion.

- It can be used to deliver all resuscitation fluids, medications and blood-derived products.

- It allows rapid adequate plasma concentration of medications similar to that of central venous administration (more rapid and reliable than that achieved through a peripheral IV).

- It allows bone marrow aspiration, which can be used for analysis. In this situation, the laboratory should be informed as the fat in a marrow sample may cause damage to auto-analysers.

Insertion of an intraosseous cannula

Before undertaking this procedure, the appropriate equipment must be available and there should be no contraindications to IO insertion (see below).

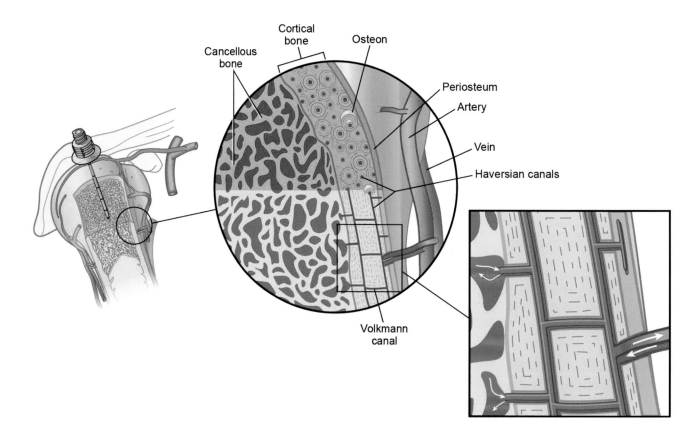

Figure 5.1 Intraosseous space and relationship with circulation

Insertion site – anatomical landmarks

The site used for IO access will vary as appropriate for the age of the patient. The insertion site of choice in infants and children is the proximal tibia with the distal tibia and distal femur as alternative access sites. With increasing age the cortical thickness of long bones, particularly the tibia increases, making penetration more difficult and requiring greater force. Therefore, in older children and adults the distal tibia or proximal humerus may be preferable, in addition these sites specifically avoid the growth plates of the bones.

Proximal tibia

The most common insertion site for IO in infants and children, because there is a flat wide surface of bone with a thin layer of overlying tissue (this allows easy identification of landmarks). Additionally the tibia is away from the airway and chest so that resuscitation efforts are not impeded by access attempts (Figure 5.2).

Landmarks – newborns, infants and small children: Insertion site is located approximately 1 cm (1 fingerbreadth) below and 1 cm (1 fingerbreadth) medial to the tibial tuberosity on the anteromedial surface of the tibia.

Landmarks – older children and adolescents: 2–3 cm below and medial to tibial tuberosity on anteromedial surface of the tibia.

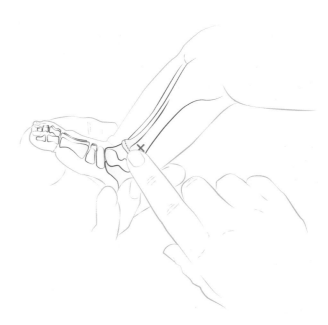

Figure 5.3 Distal tibia IO insertion landmark (X)

Distal femur

Landmarks – newborns, infants and small children only: Hold the leg straight with the knee held straight and immobilised; insert the IO needle into centro-medial aspect of the distal femur, 1–2 cm above the patella and 1–2 cm medial to the midline (Figure 5.4). The knee must remain immobilised until the IO is removed.

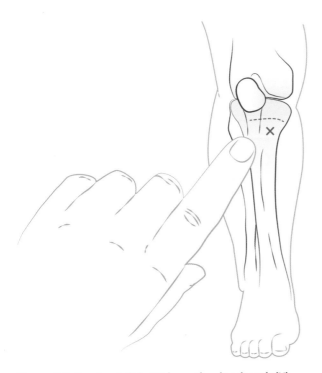

Figure 5.2 Proximal tibia IO insertion landmark (X)

Distal tibia

Landmarks – newborns, infants and small children: 1–2 cm proximal to most prominent aspect of medial malleolus.

Landmarks – older children and adolescents: 3 cm proximal to the most prominent aspect of the medial malleolus on the flat centre aspect of the bone (Figure 5.3).

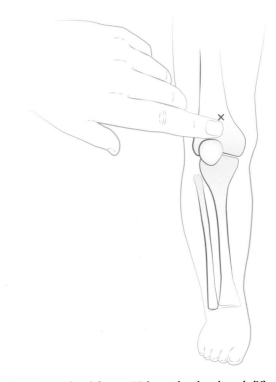

Figure 5.4 Distal femur IO insertion landmark (X)

Proximal humerus

Landmark: The greater tubercle of the humeral head. Only use in young children if landmarks can be identified and if there is pelvic and/or lower limb trauma preventing the use of the tibia. Generally, successful insertion in the humeral head requires more training and experience. To identify this landmark firstly place the patient's hand on their abdomen (to adduct the elbow and internally rotate the humerus) then place the palm of your hand over the humeral head anteriorly (it should feel like a ball and is the general area where the IO will be inserted (Figure 5.5)). Next place the ulnar aspect of your hand vertically over the axilla, then the ulnar aspect of your other hand along the midline of the upper arm laterally then join your thumbs together – this point will identify the vertical line of insertion on the proximal humerus. Feel proximally along the insertion line identifying the surgical neck of the humerus (this is where the humeral bone shaft meets the ball-like head of the humerus). The insertion site is 1–2 cm above the surgical neck on the most prominent aspect of the greater tubercle. Insert the needle using a downward angle.

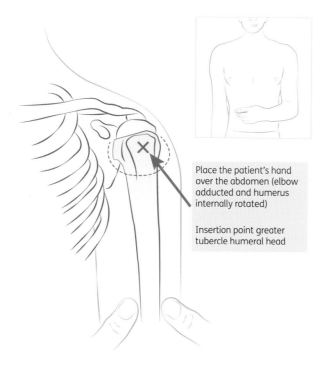

Place the patient's hand over the abdomen (elbow adducted and humerus internally rotated)

Insertion point greater tubercle humeral head

Figure 5.5 Humeral Head IO insertion landmark (X)

Contraindications

Contraindications to the insertion of an IO include osteogenesis imperfecta ('brittle bone' disease) and haemophilia or other known coagulopathies. IO cannulation should not be through an area of infected skin or wounds. Fractured bones must not be used, nor should the cannula be inserted into a bone immediately distal to a fracture site, as this may predispose to the development of compartment syndrome; similarly, if the bone has had a previous IO inserted in it within the last 48 h it should not be used.

Equipment required

1. IO cannulae:

There are IO needles intraosseous cannulae available commercially such as the Cook and Jamshidi needles (Figure 5.6) but powered needle devices such as the EZ-IO

drill (Figure 5.7) are becoming more popular. There appears to be little difference in the success rate of obtaining IO access between powered and manual devices but studies have shown that powered devices are more readily used by staff. The EZ-IO device has become the device of choice for many hospitals as it requires minimal practice and training and results show it to be a safe and rapid means of obtaining IO access. Most resuscitation trolleys should carry a manual needle as well as a powered device in case of equipment failure.

IO cannulae have a trocar and manual varieties come in a variety of sizes. Generally, it is recommended that size 18 gauge is used for a newborn-6 months of age, 16 gauge for a child between 6–18 months, and 14 gauge for children > 18 months.

The powered EZ-IO device needles are all 15 gauge but come in a variety of lengths for different ages (15, 25, 35 mm).

If there is no dedicated IO cannula available, bone marrow aspiration or spinal (lumbar puncture) needles can be used.

Additional IO cannulae should be available in case of insertion difficulties or the need to secure further vascular access (e.g. infusion of vasoactive medications; in cases of trauma where large volumes of fluid need to be rapidly infused).

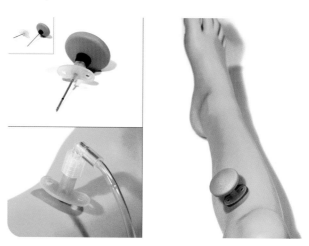

Figure 5.6 Intraosseous cannula and trocar

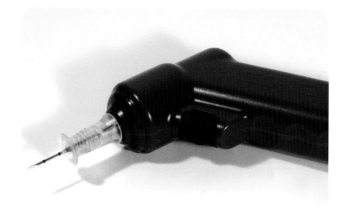

Figure 5.7 EZ-IO drill and needle

2. Alcohol-based skin preparation solution:
This minimises the risk of infection.

3. Three-way tap with integrated IV extension tubing:
This is primed with 0.9% saline and attached to a syringe also filled with 0.9% saline to minimise the risk of air emboli, confirm correct placement and allow for flushing of medications.

4. Syringe:
This is to aspirate bone marrow once the IO is inserted (e.g. to obtain a sample and/or confirm correct position).

5. Emergency medications and/or fluids:
Have these to hand to ensure prompt delivery when access is achieved.

6. Local anaesthetic agent:
If the child is still conscious, this should be considered to minimise pain along the intended track of the IO cannula. Additionally, lidocaine 1% or 2% (preservative and adrenaline FREE) may be considered for use to reduce pain associated with infusion of fluids and medications through an IO needle by local policy.

Technique for manual insertion of an IO cannula

1. Identify the site to be accessed.

2. Clean the skin around selected site with an alcohol-based solution.

3. Infiltrate the skin through to the periosteum with local anaesthetic agent (i.e. 1% lidocaine) if appropriate.

4. Immobilise the limb with your non-dominant hand ensuring no hands are placed under the limb.

5. Using your dominant hand, grasp the needle and position it at a 90° angle on the skin at the prepared site.

6. Using a firm rotating action, the needle should be advanced (approximately 1–2 cm) until loss of resistance is felt; this 'give' indicates penetration of the cortex.

7. Unscrew and withdraw the trocar.

8. The 3-way tap with integrated IV extension tubing should be attached and marrow aspirated and/or fluid flushed in to the cannula to confirm position. If it is vital to obtain a marrow sample this can be attempted at this point. However, this must not delay administration of adrenaline in cardiorespiratory arrest.

9. Rapidly flush the IO needle with at least 5–10 mL of 0.9% saline to ensure patency and check the soft tissues around the insertion site for any swelling.

10. Administer resuscitation medications and/or fluid boluses as indicated (Figure 5.8). It should be noted that, with the smaller size cannulae, a fluid bolus may be easier to deliver with a 20 mL rather than a 50 mL syringe. Pressure will be required to deliver fluids and medications as the pressure in the medullary cavity is high. A simple drip or other low pressure devices (<300 mmHg) will not be useful.

11. Fluid administration via an IO needle may be very painful in a conscious child so proper analgesia should be given using adrenaline-free 1 or 2% lidocaine.

12. Although the cannula will be stable once correctly sited, it is advisable to secure it further to prevent accidental dislodgement, particularly during transfer of the child to a definitive care facility.

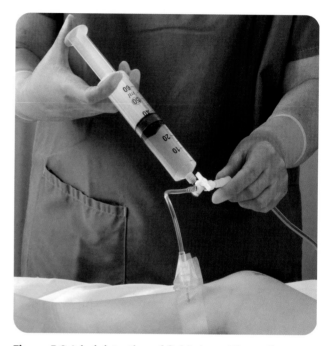

Figure 5.8 Administration of fluid via an IO needle

Complications

Although these are very uncommon, complications can occur. These include:

- Extravasation: true extravasation ('tissuing') of an IO cannula is uncommon. However, transient trivial swelling of subcutaneous tissue is commonly seen as fluid leaks from the marrow cavity into surrounding tissues. If the swelling does not rapidly subside or there is concern that the cannula is misplaced, the rescuer should withdraw a small amount of fluid; this aspirate should be blood stained if the cannula is in the correct place.

- Embolism: there is a small risk of fat or bone marrow embolism but in practice no cases have been reported.

- Infection: (e.g. osteomyelitis or cellulitis) a serious but rare complication. The risk is very low if the IO needle is removed as soon as possible.

- Compartment syndrome: which may result from a large extravasation into a fascial compartment compromising the blood supply distally; this may require surgery.

- Skin necrosis.

- Fracture.

- Damage to growth plate of epiphyses: although this is a theoretical risk no cases causing harm have been reported.

The potential for most of these complications can be minimised by removing the cannula as soon as alternative secure intravenous access has been obtained.

Central venous access

Continuous infusions of inotropes, corrosive agents (e.g. potassium) and the monitoring of central venous pressure are best performed by the central venous route. It also permits rapid infusion of large volumes of fluid, quicker onset of action and an earlier peak level of resuscitation drugs, if they are given via this route. Vasospasm and extravasation are less likely to occur with central venous than with peripheral access. However, insertion of a central venous line in a child requires training and practice and can be time-consuming (Figure 5.9).

Central venous access sites include: the right and left internal jugular veins (the right side is preferred as the vein's route is less tortuous and hence there are fewer complications), right and left subclavian veins, left and right femoral veins.

Urgent insertion of central venous line

Equipment required

- alcohol-based solution

- lidocaine 1% for local anaesthesia with a 2 mL syringe and G23 needle (in the conscious child, consider a general anaesthetic)

- syringe of 0.9% saline

- suture material

- infusion set

- adhesive tape

- over-the-needle cannula.

A G20 or larger needle should be used for rapid volume expansion and the administration of drugs. This can also be used to place a central line using a Seldinger technique.

Complications

General complications include haematoma, venous obstruction, thrombosis, thrombophlebitis, air embolism and sepsis.

Specific complications of superior vena caval access (i.e. via the subclavian or internal jugular vein) include haemothorax, pneumothorax, cardiac tamponade, arrhythmias, diaphragmatic paralysis, Horner's syndrome and puncture of the internal carotid artery.

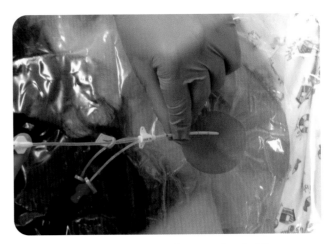

Figure 5.9 Central line placed in RIJ using Seldinger technique

Complications seen in obtaining inferior vena cava access (i.e. via the femoral vein) include intestinal perforation, haematoma of the inguinal or retroperitoneal areas, septic arthritis of the hip and renal vein thrombosis.

Femoral vein

The inguinal site is most commonly used during cardiopulmonary resuscitation as its distance from the head and chest allows cannulation without interrupting the management of the airway and breathing. This is a technique best carried out by the experienced clinician.

Technique

1. Place the leg in slight external rotation.

2. Clean the skin at the site of insertion.

3. Identify the puncture site. The vein is directly medial to the femoral artery. If the artery is not palpable, its location corresponds to the point midway between the anterior superior iliac spine and the pubic symphysis. During chest compressions pulsations should be felt in the femoral artery.

4. If the child is aware of pain, lidocaine 1% should be used to infiltrate the puncture site. General anaesthesia should be considered in the conscious child.

5. Attach the cannula with a needle to a saline-filled syringe, introduce it at a 45° angle, pointing the bevel of the needle towards the child's head, directly over the vein and keep the syringe in line with the child's thigh.

6. Advance the needle, pulling back on the plunger once the needle is below the surface of the skin.

7. As soon as blood flows back into the syringe, stop advancing it.

8. Gently remove the needle with the syringe, leaving the cannula in the vein.

9. Occlude the end of the cannula to prevent blood loss.

10. Confirm the location of the cannula by attempting to aspirate blood and, if blood is obtained, flush the cannula with 0.9% saline and attach it to a pre-flushed 3-way tap.

11. Generally it is safer if the catheter is sutured in place.

Fluid administration for volume resuscitation

Intravascular fluids are primarily administered to restore circulatory volume and ensure adequate perfusion of vital organs.

During cardiorespiratory arrest, hypovolaemia is often a primary contributory factor and fluid resuscitation may play a critical part in achieving return of spontaneous circulation (ROSC).

The administration of fluids is also indicated for any child exhibiting signs of circulatory failure (e.g. decreased skin perfusion, prolonged capillary refill time, hypotension). Caution is advised in children and infants with suspected cardiogenic shock where the heart is unable to deal with the volume load or those with diabetic ketoacidosis when large fluids shifts are undesirable (Chapter 10).

Fluid volumes

There has been much debate about the appropriate size of fluid bolus volume for resuscitation in children following a large study in a number of African countries which suggested that aggressive fluid administration may worsen outcome. The application of this study to children treated in more advanced health care systems is not known but should prompt all healthcare providers to carefully assess the effect of each fluid bolus on the child's clinical condition. Use a cautious approach to fluid therapy in children with febrile illness who do not have any signs of circulatory failure.

During the resuscitation of a child with compromised circulation due to hypovolaemia (including sepsis and anaphylaxis), initial resuscitation fluid is administered as a bolus of 20 mL kg^{-1} of isotonic fluid. **The child's circulatory status should then be reassessed** and if signs of circulatory failure persist, this should be repeated. **Re-assessment after each fluid bolus** is important to try and prevent over transfusion of fluid; signs of overload include moist sounds ('crackles') at the lung bases, jugular venous distension in children and/or liver distension in infants.

If there is no improvement in circulatory status following 40–60 mL kg^{-1}, ongoing losses must be suspected (e.g. diarrhoeal fluid, bleeding). The aim in the management of hypovolaemic shock is to prevent the onset of decompensated circulatory failure, as this may lead to irreversible cardiorespiratory failure and death.

In septic shock, fluid resuscitation is specifically required as vasodilatation may be considerable and there may be a relatively hypovolaemic state. Up to 60–80 mL kg^{-1} of volume expansion is often required in the first hour of resuscitation; larger volumes (> 100 mL kg^{-1}) can be required within the first few hours. Inotropes (and intubation) may also be required in children with septic shock and should be considered at an early stage (e.g. after 40 mL kg^{-1}). Call for senior help early as intubation is safer when cardiovascular stability has been achieved.

Fluids must be infused during cardiorespiratory arrest if hypovolaemic shock is a likely cause of the arrest. However, excessive amounts of fluid may be harmful in cardiac arrest with other causes and in post-resuscitation states. Measurement of blood pressure (BP) is of little help in determining circulatory status as it remains normal in compensated circulatory failure and only starts to drop as decompensation develops.

Circulatory failure without hypovolaemia: if circulatory failure is due to other causes, such as cardiac failure, a smaller initial volume (10 mL kg^{-1}) should be used. The effect of each smaller bolus should be carefully assessed to ensure that fluid administration is not causing worsening of the circulation (e.g. appearance of crackles at the lung bases and increasing size of liver edge). In some patients with cardiac failure diuretics such as furosemide may be indicated for fluid overload.

Fluid bolus in trauma: initial fluid bolus size should be 10 mL kg^{-1} 0.9% saline with careful re-assessment after each bolus. If the child is haemorrhaging consider blood and blood products for third and subsequent boluses guided by bedside, point of care, haemoglobin (Hb) measurement. An exception would be for children with massive haemorrhage on presentation when blood would immediately be given and the massive transfusion protocol activated. Over-transfusion is not desirable and may add to morbidity so careful reassessment and haemoglobin measurements are required. Most children with traumatic injuries have head injuries and it is ***extremely important*** to maintain a good blood pressure to support cerebral perfusion. Surgical referral should be made for full patient evaluation as haemostasis may only be achieved by surgery. The principles of management adhere to the ABCDE (airway, breathing, circulation, disability, exposure) approach with fluid administration forming part of the 'C' phase of resuscitation.

Types of fluid

In the initial phase of resuscitation, isotonic salt solutions should be used (isotonic means that the solution used has a similar sodium concentration as that in the plasma). There are no clear advantages between using crystalloid or colloid solutions. Glucose containing solutions (such as dextrose-saline) should never be used for volume replacement as they can cause hyponatraemia (which can cause seizures) and hyperglycaemia, which in turn, can lead to further fluid loss.

Crystalloids

Examples of appropriate resuscitation crystalloids include:

- 0.9% saline

- Ringer's lactate

- Hartmann's solution

- Plasmalyte.

Crystalloids are cheap, readily available and do not cause allergic reactions. They are, however, marginally less efficient than colloids at increasing circulating volume within the intravascular space, as they rapidly move into the surrounding interstitium; only 50–75% of the administered volume remains in the intravascular compartment. Therefore, to correct the initial circulatory deficit volume, 1.5–2 times this volume has to be infused; this may be poorly tolerated in children with underlying cardiac or respiratory disease, and pulmonary oedema may occur.

Crystalloids are indicated to replace fluid loss from the interstitial space and to correct electrolyte deficiencies, as seen in patients with burns or those who are dehydrated.

Large quantities of saline, but not Ringer's lactate, may induce hyperchloraemic acidosis (which some studies suggest *may* cause additional morbidity by affecting renal and immune function), therefore monitoring of the blood electrolyte concentrations should occur. Bolus infusion of fluids containing potassium must be avoided during resuscitation, (particularly important in children with anuria or oliguria, as hyperkalaemia could arise).

Glucose solutions should never be used for volume expansion as they can cause hyperglycaemia, resulting in osmotic diuresis. This increases urine production and so increases circulatory volume loss. Glucose solutions should only be used to correct hypoglycaemia following measurement of blood sugar levels: 2 mL kg^{-1} of 10% glucose is given and the patient's blood sugar should be re-measured shortly afterwards to ensure it is within the normal range. In the newborn 2.5 mL kg^{-1} of 10% glucose may be given during resuscitation at birth to correct hypoglycaemia.

Colloids

Examples of colloids include:

- Human albumin (4.5%) solution

- Fresh frozen plasma (FFP)

- Gelatin solutions (e.g. Gelofusin).

Colloids are relatively expensive and less readily available than crystalloids. Colloids should not be used in anaphylaxis because of the potential risk of allergic reaction. The main reason for considering the use of colloids in resuscitation is that they remain in the vascular space for longer, and may therefore increase the circulatory volume more efficiently than crystalloids, although the effect is far less than previously assumed.

Starch solutions are not used in children and infants as they cause detrimental effects on renal function, coagulation and mortality.

Blood products

The administration of blood products is reserved for situations where there is a specific indication for their use (i.e. blood loss or coagulopathy). If the infusion of 20 mL kg^{-1} (i.e. 10 mL kg^{-1} bolus x 2) does not improve the circulatory status of a child who has suffered trauma, transfusion of blood must be considered, as well as urgent surgical referral. In an emergency, Group O Rhesus-negative 'flying squad' blood or type-specific uncross-matched blood may be used for transfusion until fully cross-matched blood is available. If a trauma patient has required > 40 mL kg^{-1} of blood the massive transfusion protocol should be activated so that there is replacement of other blood products in addition to red cells (Chapter 11).

Fresh frozen plasma should only be used in resuscitation situations for the treatment of coagulation abnormalities, or as part of a massive transfusion protocol. Other blood products (e.g. cryoprecipitate and platelets) are usually given based on the findings of laboratory or near patient testing.

Although blood products are now very safe, the risks of blood product administration must always be considered.

First-line resuscitation medications

Only a few medications are indicated during the initial resuscitation phase of a child in cardiorespiratory arrest. Administration of medications should be considered only after adequate ventilation and chest compressions have been established, and in the case of a shockable arrhythmia (VF or pulseless pVT), following delivery of the first three defibrillation shocks.

For safety reasons, as well as speed and ease of use, the use of pre-filled medication syringes is advocated.

All medications administered should be followed by a flush of 2–5 mL 0.9% saline to ensure they reach the circulation and to minimise the risks of interactions with any other medications or fluids given via the same cannula. All medications and fluids should be recorded as they are administered and then documented at the end of the resuscitation attempt.

Adrenaline

Indications for use:

- cardiorespiratory arrest of any aetiology

- bradycardia < 60 min^{-1} with decompensated circulatory shock after the initial steps to restore satisfactory oxygenation and ventilation have been taken

- first line inotrope as an infusion centrally or peripherally in fluid resistant septic shock.

- hypotension with anaphylaxis.

In cardiac arrest with non shockable rhythms adrenaline should be given as soon as circulatory access has been achieved, as early administration is associated with better outcomes. In shockable rhythms adrenaline should be given after the third defibrillation and then following alternate shocks thereafter (following 3rd shock then following 5th shock etc).

Dosage: in cardiorespiratory arrest or bradycardia with decompensated circulatory failure 10 mcg kg^{-1} (or 0.1 mL kg^{-1} of 1:10 000 solution). This is repeated every 3–5 min as necessary.

Actions: adrenaline is an endogenous, directly acting sympathomimetic amine with both alpha and beta adrenergic activity. In the dose used in resuscitation, adrenaline produces vasoconstriction, which results in increased cerebral and coronary perfusion pressure. It also increases myocardial contractility and may facilitate defibrillation success.

Alpha adrenergic effects cause splanchnic and mucocutaneous vasoconstriction with increased systolic and diastolic blood pressure. Beta-1 and 2 adrenergic effects increase the force and rate of myocardial contractions, and cause vascular smooth muscle vasodilatation and bronchiolar smooth muscle relaxation. Adrenaline's pharmacological effects are dose-related.

In cardiorespiratory arrest, alpha adrenergic-mediated vasoconstriction is the most important pharmacological action of adrenaline as this increases the diastolic pressure, so enhancing coronary perfusion and oxygen delivery to the heart. This is a critical determinant for successful resuscitation.

Other beneficial effects include:

- elevation of systolic BP

- increased tendency for a normal cardiac perfusing rhythm to develop during cardiorespiratory resuscitation

- enhanced contractile state of the heart and stimulated spontaneous cardiac contractions

- increased intensity of ventricular fibrillation, so increasing the likelihood of successful response to defibrillation (i.e. return to normal rhythm).

The most commonly observed rhythms in the paediatric patient with cardiorespiratory arrest are asystole and bradyarrhythmia; adrenaline may generate a perfusing rhythm in these children. As the action of catecholamines may be depressed by acidosis pay careful attention to oxygenation, ventilation and circulation is essential (i.e. ABCDE).

Catecholamines are inactivated by alkaline solutions and should never be given simultaneously with sodium bicarbonate via the same vascular access cannula. If only one cannula is available and both these medications are to be used, their administration must be separated by a bolus of 0.9% saline (2–5 mL).

Asystole, pulseless electrical activity (PEA), ventricular fibrillation (VF) and pulseless ventricular tachycardia (pVT) all require the same dosage regime, 10 mcg kg^{-1} of adrenaline (or 0.1 mL kg^{-1} of a 1: 10 000 solution (1 mg 10 mL^{-1})) by IV or IO route. Adrenaline is given every 3–5 min (or every two loops of 2 min of CPR), starting after the third defibrillation for the shockable rhythm protocol.

In newborns, the maximum dose is 10–30 mcg kg^{-1} (or 0.1–0.3 mL kg^{-1} of a 1:10 000 solution) by IV or IO route. The tracheal route is not recommended. Large doses of adrenaline may increase the risk of intracranial haemorrhage in newborns, especially in preterm infants.

The half-life of adrenaline is short (2 min) and doses are repeated until the desired effect is achieved; hence, a continuous infusion of adrenaline may occasionally be necessary once spontaneous circulation is restored.

The haemodynamic effects are dose-related:

- Low-dose infusions (< 0.1 mcg kg^{-1} min^{-1}) produce beta-adrenergic effects

- High-dose infusions (> 0.1 mcg kg^{-1} min^{-1}) produce alpha-adrenergic mediated vasoconstriction.

Precaution: boluses of adrenaline should be administered via a secure vascular (IV or IO) cannula. If ongoing post-resuscitation care requires an adrenaline infusion, this should be through a central venous cannula when possible.

Adrenaline frequently causes tachycardia and may produce or exacerbate ventricular ectopics.

Higher doses of adrenaline administered by any route are not recommended as they do not improve survival or neurological outcome after cardiorespiratory arrest although they may be required in exceptional circumstances (e.g. adrenoceptor blocker overdose).

Adenosine

Adenosine is an endogenous purine nucleoside causing atrioventricular block of very short duration. It impairs accessory bundle re-entry at the atrioventricular node (AV). This accessory bundle is responsible for most supraventricular tachycardia (SVT) in children.

Adenosine is rapidly metabolised by red blood cells and its half-life is only 10 s. Therefore, it should be injected rapidly and as close to the heart as possible (via a central or upper limb peripheral intravenous route) and immediately followed by a rapid bolus of 0.9% saline.

Side effects (flushing, headache, hypotension, bronchospasm, anxiety and a sense of impending doom) are short-lived, owing to its short half-life.

Indication for use: adenosine is used in management of SVT as it impairs accessory bundle re-entry at the AV node.

Dosage: 100 mcg kg^{-1} IV or IO bolus (maximum dose 6 mg) is rapidly followed by 3–5 mL of 0.9% saline. The second dose may be doubled (maximum 12 mg). Continuous cardiac monitoring is required to interpret the initial rhythm and monitor the effect of adenosine, which may be diagnostic.

Precautions: children treated with theophylline are less sensitive to the effects of adenosine. Adenosine should be used with caution in asthmatics (as it can invoke severe bronchospasm) and children who have undergone a heart transplant.

Amiodarone

Indication for use: refractory VF or pVT. If VF or pVT persists after the third defibrillation, a dose of amiodarone should be given with adrenaline. This can be repeated after the fifth shock if defibrillation is still unsuccessful.

Dosage: 5 mg kg^{-1}.

Actions: amiodarone is a membrane-stabilising anti-arrhythmic medication that increases the duration of the action potential and refractory period in both atrial and ventricular myocardium.

> Atrioventricular conduction is also slowed, and a similar effect is seen in accessory pathways. Amiodarone has a mild negative inotropic action and causes peripheral vasodilatation through non-competitive alpha-blocking effects. The hypotension that occurs with IV amiodarone is related to the rate of delivery and is due more to the solvent (Polysorbate 80 and benzyl alcohol), which causes histamine release, than the drug itself. The oral form is not well absorbed but the intravenous form has been successfully used for tachyarrhythmia management.

Precaution: amiodarone should be given as a pre-filled syringe preparation or diluted in 5% glucose. Ideally, it should be administered via a central vascular (IV or IO) route as it can cause thrombophlebitis. If it has to be given peripherally it should be liberally flushed with 0.9% saline .

In the treatment of shockable rhythms, give an initial IV bolus dose of amiodarone 5 mg kg^{-1} after the third shock. Repeat the dose after the fifth shock if still in VF/pVT.

If defibrillation was successful but VF/pVT recurs, amiodarone can be repeated (unless two doses have already been injected) in which case a continuous infusion should be started.

In SVT, amiodarone must be injected slowly (over 20–60 min) to avoid hypotension. Systemic BP and ECG should be continuously monitored.

Other rare but significant adverse effects are bradycardia and polymorphic ventricular tachycardia.

Atropine

Indication for use: bradycardia resulting from vagal stimulation. There is no evidence that atropine has any benefit in asphyxial bradycardia or asystole and its routine use has been removed from the advanced life support algorithms.

Dosage: 20 mcg kg^{-1}.

This dose may be repeated but, once the vagus nerve has been fully blocked, there is no further beneficial effect. Until recently a minimum dose of 100 mcg was recommended as there was thought to be a paradoxical bradycardia with lower doses but recent data does not support this so 20 mcg kg^{-1} doses are acceptable in babies weighing less than 5 kg.

Actions: atropine blocks the effect of the vagus nerve on the sinoatrial (SA) and atrioventricular (AV) nodes, increasing sinus automaticity, facilitating AV node conduction and increasing heart rate. The functions of the vagus nerve include pupillary constriction, contraction of the gut and production of salivary and gastro-intestinal secretions. During resuscitation, atropine may be of benefit in treating bradycardia which accompanies actions that result in vagal stimulation such as laryngoscopy.

Sodium bicarbonate

This is not a first-line resuscitation medication. Studies have shown that the routine use of sodium bicarbonate does not improve outcome.

Indication for use: It may be considered in prolonged arrest and it has a specific role in management of hyperkalaemia and the arrhythmias associated with tricyclic antidepressants.

Dosage: the initial dose is 1 mmol kg^{-1}. This equates to 1 mL kg^{-1} of 8.4% solution, although in newborns and infants < 3 months the weaker concentration (i.e. 4.2%) solution should be used to limit the osmotic load.

The decision to give further doses should be based on blood gas analysis.

Actions: sodium bicarbonate is administered to reverse metabolic acidosis. However, as it elevates $PaCO_2$ levels, the administration of sodium bicarbonate may worsen existing respiratory acidosis, a possible cause of the cardiorespiratory arrest. It may also cause paradoxical intracellular acidosis, thus worsening cellular function (e.g. myocardial dysfunction may be induced by the acidosis within myocardial cells). Some of the specific effects of sodium bicarbonate administration include:

- carbon dioxide production which diffuses into cells and exacerbates the intracellular acidosis

- left displacement of the oxyhaemoglobin dissociation curve inhibiting oxygen release to the tissues

- intracellular shift of potassium

- hypernatraemia due to the high, osmotically active, sodium content

- lowered VF threshold

- decreased plasma calcium.

The potential negative effects of sodium bicarbonate outweigh any benefits unless the metabolic acidosis is severe, and even then it should be used with caution.

Precautions: arterial blood gas analysis does not reflect venous or tissue pH and should be interpreted with caution. Care should also be taken to ensure that an adequate flush of 0.9% saline is given between delivery of sodium bicarbonate and any other medications via the same cannula, as incompatibilities may occur.

Calcium

Calcium is essential to myocardial contraction. However its routine administration does not improve the outcome of cardiorespiratory arrest. High plasma concentrations achieved after injection may be harmful to the ischaemic myocardium and may also impair cerebral recovery. After ischaemia and during reperfusion of ischaemic organs cytoplasmic calcium would appear to contribute to cellular necrosis. The administration of calcium during cardiorespiratory arrest has been associated with increased mortality.

Indication for use: routine administration of calcium in advanced life support is not recommended. It is only indicated for the treatment of documented hypocalcaemia, hyperkalaemia, hypermagnesaemia and overdose of calcium channel blockers. Hypocalcaemia is frequently seen in septic patients who need repeated fluid boluses or trauma patients needing multiple blood transfusions.

Dosage: 0.2 mL kg^{-1} of 10% calcium chloride.

Precautions: rapid calcium injection may induce bradyarrhythmia and asystole in patients treated with digoxin. The dose should be infused by slow injection via central intravenous access, as calcium may produce chemical burns if it leaks into surrounding tissues.

Glucose

Indication for use: documented hypoglycaemia. Neonatal, child and adult data show that both hyper- and hypo-glycaemia are associated with worse outcomes after cardiorespiratory arrest. Plasma glucose concentrations should be monitored closely in any ill or injured child, including after cardiorespiratory arrest. Do not give glucose-containing fluids during CPR except for the treatment of hypoglycaemia. Hyper- and hypo-glycaemia should be avoided following ROSC but tight glucose control

has not shown survival benefits when compared with moderate glucose control in adults or children and increased the risk of hypoglycaemia.

Infants have high glucose requirements and low glycogen storage. They can readily become hypoglycaemic during coma, circulatory and respiratory failure. It is therefore necessary to monitor closely their blood glucose concentrations.

The clinical signs of hypoglycaemia and shock may have similarities, (i.e. hypotension, tachycardia, decreased peripheral perfusion and sweating). Additionally children and infants with hypoglycaemia may present with coma and or seizures.

Dosage: 200 mg kg^{-1} (or 2 mL kg^{-1}) of 10% glucose solution.

Newborn 2.5 mL kg^{-1} of 10% glucose solution

Re-checking the blood glucose value should be performed shortly afterwards (e.g. 2 min following administration) to determine if further dosages are required.

Actions: glucose is a principal energy substrate of all body tissues including the brain and myocardial cells. Low blood levels mean that myocardial contractility and therefore cardiac output, may be reduced.

Precaution: the association between hypoglycaemia and seizures is well documented. Prevention of seizures is essential to minimise the risk of neurological insult. Additionally, studies have shown a correlation between poor neurological outcome and hyperglycaemia. It is therefore important that blood glucose measurement is repeated regularly to ensure it is maintained within the normal range.

Once resuscitation has been completed, a continuous infusion of a glucose-containing solution is preferable to serial bolus therapy with hypertonic glucose. Repeated hyperglycaemia may increase serum osmolarity with the risk of osmotic diuresis. There is also a risk of intraventricular haemorrhage in the premature neonate if bolus(es) of hypertonic solutions is/are used. A risk of cutaneous necrosis exists if hypertonic glucose leaks into surrounding tissues.

Magnesium

This is a major intracellular cation and serves as a co-factor in many enzymatic reactions. Magnesium treatment is indicated in children with documented hypomagnesaemia or with polymorphic VT (torsade de pointes), regardless of cause.

Dosage: 0.5 mL kg^{-1} 10% magnesium sulfate repeated as necessary.

Magnesium may also be a useful drug in the treatment of acute asthma as it causes smooth muscle relaxation.

Naloxone

Naloxone is a fast acting (2 min after injection) opiate antagonist with duration of action up to 45 min. In cases of overdose with drugs such as methadone which has a slow-release form, continuous naloxone infusion may be required to counteract further effects of the opiate.

Indication for use: symptomatic opiate poisoning. Clinical signs include respiratory depression, coma, pupillary constriction (miosis), hypotension and decreased perfusion.

Dosage: the recommended initial dose for full reversal of opiate effects is 100 mcg kg^{-1} in children under five years (maximum 2 mg) and 2 mg in those over five years, administered via IV, IO or intramuscular route. If necessary, naloxone can be repeated every 3 min.Titrated smaller doses can be used to partially reverse opiate effect, where full reversal may result in extreme pain, for example in a drowsy post-operative patient with a low respiratory rate.

A continuous naloxone infusion may be used if it is suspected that the patient has received a large amount of opiates. The infusion can range between 10–160 mcg kg^{-1} h^{-1} and is titrated until a satisfactory sustained response is obtained.

Precautions: serious complications after naloxone treatment are uncommon (< 2%). However, if used for abrupt withdrawal from opiates, severe complications have been described (e.g. seizures, pulmonary oedema, ventricular arrhythmia and hypertension).

Dopamine: *Dopamine is a catecholamine that may be used as an inotrope (a drug increasing the force of cardiac contraction) in paediatric sepsis, however it is no longer a first line choice. It can be given centrally as an intravenous infusion. In the dose range 5–10 mcg kg^{-1} min^{-1} beta adrenergic agonist effects predominate with increased cardiac index (CI) and increased heart rate. At doses > 10 mcg kg^{-1} min^{-1} alpha adrenergic agonist effects occur with vasoconstriction and subsequent increased systemic vascular resistance (SVR) and further increases in heart rate.*

Furosemide: *is a loop diuretic which binds to a sodium transporter in the ascending loop of Henle in the kidney. This results in an increase of sodium and hence water lost in the urine. Furosemide is useful in reducing the intravascular fluid volume in fluid overload states and in cardiac failure.*

Ketamine: *is a potent sedative, amnesic, analgesic and anaesthetic agent. It can provide anaesthesia and sedation with relatively less effect on respiratory drive and maintains protective airway reflexes. Ketamine also has a relatively stable haemodynamic profile as it blocks re-uptake of catecholamines so it may be beneficial in intubation in septic shock.*

Lidocaine: *is a commonly used anaesthetic agent and a class 1b anti-arrhythmic drug. Lidocaine is an alternative to amiodarone in defibrillation resistant VF/pVT; loading dose 1 mg kg^{-1} (maximum 100 mg) followed by an infusion of 20–50 mcg kg^{-1} min^{-1}. Toxicity can occur if there is underlying renal or hepatic disease.*

Lorazepam: *is a benzodiazepine with anti-seizure, sedation and amnesic properties. It is a longer acting and more potent anti-convulsant than diazepam. It is given intravenously when the seizure has been > 5 min long in a dose of 0.1 mg kg^{-1} this can repeated if no effect after 10 min.*

Milrinone: *Is a type 3 phosphodiesterase inhibitor which potentiates the effects of beta receptor stimulation in cardiac and vascular tissue resulting in increased inotrope effect (increased force of cardiac contraction) and peripheral vasodilatation (which can cause hypotension). Milrinone may also have other beneficial effects on cardiac function and can be used in septic shock.*

Noradrenaline: *is a catecholamine with predominantly alpha 1 adrenergic agonist effects resulting in increased SVR and BP with less effect on heart rate. It is useful in management of septic shock particularly warm shock.*

Phenobarbital: *is a barbiturate which increases GABA activity in the brain and depresses glutamate activity; the overall effect is to decrease CNS electrical activity hence its effectiveness in seizures. It can also cause sedation, respiratory depression and hypotension particularly in combination with benzodiazepines.*

Phenytoin: *is a membrane stabilising drug which inhibits the spread of seizure activity in the motor cortex. It is used in the status epilepticus algorithm if benzodiazepines have failed to terminate seizures. It must be given slowly intravenously as it can cause profound bradycardia, hypotension, cardiac arrhythmia and even asystole.*

Salbutamol: *This has a beta 2 agonist effect relaxing smooth muscle in the airways of patients with asthma. It is sometimes also used in the treatment of hyperkalaemia.*

Vasopressin: *This has been successfully used to increase SVR in patients resistant to noradrenaline.*

Summary learning

- Intraosseous access is the circulatory route of choice in cardiorespiratory arrest and decompensated circulatory failure.
- Fluid resuscitation for hypovolaemia starts with 20 mL kg^{-1} boluses.
- After each fluid bolus, the child's condition must be reassessed.
- The role of medications is secondary to effective ventilation and chest compressions (and defibrillation where indicated) in the management of cardiorespiratory arrest.
- The main medication used in cardiorespiratory arrest is IV or IO adrenaline, which can be repeated as necessary every 3–5 min.
- Amiodarone is used in refractory VF or pVT after the third and fifth shock.
- Hypoglycaemia and hyperglycaemia should be avoided.

My key take-home messages from this chapter

Further reading

Sarisoy O, Balaogh K, Tugay S, Barn E, Gokalp AS. Efficacy of magnesium sulphate for treatment of ventricular tachycardia in Amitriptyline overdose. Paediatric Emergency care 2007; 23: 9, 646-648.

Dauchot P, Gravenstein JS. Effects of atropine on the electrocardiogram in different age groups. Clin Pharmacol Ther 1971;12:274-80.

Griesdale DE, de Souza RJ, van Dam RM, et al. Intensive insulin therapy and mortality among critically ill patients: a meta-analysis including NICE-SUGAR study data. CMAJ 2009;180:821-7.

Wiener RS, Wiener DC, Larson RJ. Benefits and risks of tight glucose control in critically ill adults: a meta-analysis. JAMA 2008;300:933-44.

Krinsley JS, Grover A. Severe hypoglycemia in critically ill patients: risk factors and outcomes. Crit Care Med 2007;35:2262-7.

Padkin A. Glucose control after cardiac arrest. Resuscitation 2009;80:611-2.

Brenner T, Bernhard M, Helm M et al. Comparison of two Intraosseous systems for adult emergency use. Resuscitation 2008; 78: 3, 314-319.

Nadkarni VM, Larkin GL, Peberdy MA, Carey SM, Kaye W, Mancini ME, et al. First documented rhythm and clinical outcome from in-hospital cardiac arrest among children and adults. JAMA. 2006 Jan 4;295(1):50-7.

Finfer S, Bellomo R, Boyce N, French J, Myburgh J, Norton R. A comparison of albumin and saline for fluid resuscitation in the intensive care unit. N Engl J Med. 2004 May 27;350(22):2247-56.

Dumas F, Dumas F, Bougouin W, Geri G, et al. Is Epinephrine During Cardiac Arrest Associated With Worse Outcomes in Resuscitated Patients? J Am Coll Cardiol. 2014;64(22):2360-2367.

Hagihara A, Hasegawa M, Abe T, Nagata T, Wakata Y, Miyazaki S. Prehospital Epinephrine Use and Survival Among Patients With Out-of-Hospital Cardiac Arrest; JAMA 21 March 2012, Vol 307, No. 11, pp 1161-1168;

Santhanam I, Sangareddi S, Venkataraman S, Kissoon N, Thiruvengadamudayan V, Kasthuri RK. A prospective randomized controlled study of two fluid regimens in the initial management of septic shock in the emergency department. Pediatr Emerg Care. 2008 Oct; 24 (10):647-55.

Maitland K, Kiguli S, Opoka RO, Engoru C, Olupot-Olupot P, Akech SO, Nyeko R, Mtove G, Reyburn H, Lang T, Brent B, Evans JA, Tibenderana JK, Crawley J, Russell EC, Levin M, Babiker AG, Gibb DM; FEAST Trial Group. Mortality after fluid bolus in African children with severe infection. NEJM. 2011, Jun 30;364(26):2483-95.

Valdes SO, Donoghue AJ, Hoyme DB, Hammond R, Berg MD, Berg RA, Samson RA; American Heart Association Get With The Guidelines-Resuscitation Investigators.. Outcomes associated with amiodarone and lidocaine in the treatment of in-hospital paediatric cardiac arrest with pulseless ventricular tachycardia or ventricular fibrillation. Resuscitation 2014, Mar;85(3):381-6.

Eisa L et al. Do small doses of atropine (< 0.1 mg) cause bradycardia in young children? Arch Dis Child 2015;100:684-8.

Andersen LW, Berg KM, Saindon BZ et al. Time to Epinephrine and Survival After Pediatric In-Hospital Cardiac Arrest. JAMA 2015;314(8):802-810.

EPALS

Rhythm recognition

Contents

- **ECG monitoring**
- **Abnormal ECG traces and clinical correlation**
- **How to manage the common tachycardia and bradycardia arrhythmias seen in acutely unwell children**

Learning outcomes

To enable you to:

- **Describe the normal electrocardiogram (ECG) trace**
- **Recognise cardiac rhythms associated with cardiorespiratory arrest**
- **Discuss the management of bradycardia**
- **Differentiate between sinus tachycardia (ST) and supraventricular tachycardia (SVT)**
- **Consider the management priorities in children with compensated and decompensated tachyarrhythmias**

ECG monitoring

Once optimal ventilation and oxygenation have been established, all seriously ill children should have their ECG monitored continuously via lead II and at least one 12-lead ECG should be performed. This facilitates the observation of heart rate and rhythm changes, which are important indicators of the response to treatments, or the evolution of the disease process. Normal heart rates vary for physiological reasons (e.g. pain, pyrexia and wakefulness), and with age (Table 6.1).

Table 6.1: Heart rate ranges (beats min⁻¹)			
Age	Mean	Awake	Deep sleep
Newborn – 3 months	140	85–205	80–140
3 months – 2 years	130	100–180	75–160
2 – 10 years	80	60–140	60–90
> 10 years	75	60–100	50–90

Acute illness in children can result in cardiac arrhythmias. Less frequently, the cardiac arrhythmia may be the precipitant for the episode of acute illness. In these cases there is commonly an underlying cardiac anatomic anomaly or reason for electrolyte disturbance causing abnormal cardiac electrical conductivity.

Examples include:

- acquired cardiac disease (e.g. cardiomyopathy, myocarditis)

- congenital heart disease or following cardiac surgery

- electrolyte disturbances (e.g. renal disease).

Additionally, some medications in therapeutic or toxic amounts may also cause arrhythmias (e.g. digoxin, beta-blockers, tricyclic antidepressants).

By monitoring the ECG, it is possible to detect those arrhythmias that are (or have the potential to become) life-threatening.

Basic electrocardiography

The ECG trace represents electrical activity within the heart, not the effectiveness of myocardial contraction or tissue perfusion. The child's clinical status needs to be considered alongside the ECG trace: **treat the patient** not the monitor.

When evaluating the ECG, possible artefacts may occur; detachment of ECG electrodes or leads can simulate asystole, whilst vibrations transmitted to the leads (e.g. during patient transportation) can mimic ventricular fibrillation (VF).

A normal ECG complex consists of a P wave, a QRS complex and a T wave (Figure 6.1).

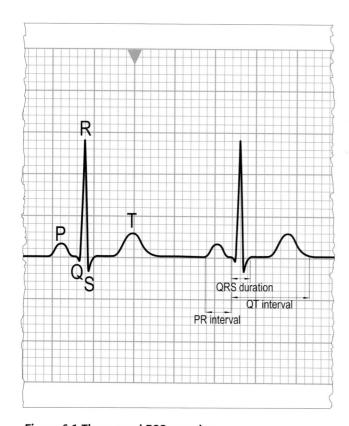

Figure 6.1 The normal ECG complex

The P wave represents electrical depolarisation of the atria. The time taken for depolarisation to pass through the atria, atrio-ventricular (AV) node and His-Purkinje system to the ventricles (Figure 6.2) is represented by the P-R interval. The QRS complex represents depolarisation of the ventricles. The ST segment and the T wave represent ventricular repolarisation, in preparation for the next impulse. A prolonged QT interval (a delay between the beginning of ventricular depolarisation and repolarisation) is a risk factor for arrhythmias and sudden death.

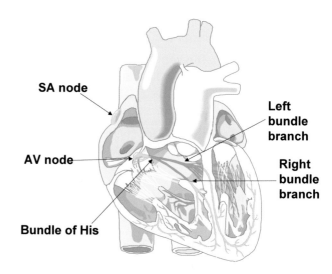

Figure 6.2 Electrical conduction through the heart

Cardiac rhythm disturbances

The approach to managing a child with a cardiac rhythm disturbance is summarised in Figure 6.3. This approach is based on determining the following four factors:

1. Presence or absence of circulation (i.e. a central pulse and other 'signs of life').

2. Clinical status – compensated (haemodynamically stable) or decompenstated (haemodynamically unstable).

3. Heart rate (bradycardia or tachycardia).

4. Width of QRS complexes on ECG (i.e. narrow or broad).

1. Presence of central pulse

Adopt the ABCDE approach and quickly establish the absence or presence of cardiac output (i.e. 'signs of life' and a palpable central pulse).

Absent pulse

The absence of 'signs of life' and no palpable central pulse indicates cardiorespiratory arrest. BLS should be started immediately. The rhythms associated with cardiorespiratory arrest are:

- asystole (or severe bradycardia)

- pulseless electrical activity (PEA)

- ventricular fibrillation (VF)

- pulseless ventricular tachycardia (pVT).

The commonest cardiorespiratory arrest arrhythmia in paediatrics is asystole (generally preceded by progressive bradycardia). The term PEA describes the situation where there is organised electrical activity displayed on the ECG monitor but no cardiac output. The principles of managing both asystole and PEA are the provision of effective CPR, early administration of adrenaline and the treatment of any underlying problems.

Both VF and pVT are less common in children, but more likely in those with underlying cardiac disease. The priority of management in these arrhythmias is effective CPR and rapid defibrillation. VF and pVT may also occur as a secondary rhythm during reperfusion of the myocardium during a cardiorespiratory arrest.

The management of cardiorespiratory arrest arrhythmias is outlined in Chapter 8.

Pulse present

If there is a central pulse present, determine whether or not the child is compensated (haemodynamically stable) or decompensated (haemodynamically unstable).

2. Clinical status

Compensated circulatory failure

The child with compensated circulatory failure, who is conscious and haemodynamically stable, must be monitored, including an ECG. If the ECG displays an arrhythmia, the child may need treatment, but it is reasonable to await expert help such as from a paediatric cardiologist. Preparations should be made to intervene (along the principles described below) should the child deteriorate and become decompensated.

Decompensated circulatory failure

The child who is decompensated (haemodynamically unstable) should be monitored and, if the ECG displays a life-threatening arrhythmia, the immediate interventions that may be required are outlined below. Urgent expert help must also be sought. This should include an anaesthetist as sedation or anaesthesia may be required to manage a conscious child requiring cardioversion.

3. Heart rate

Both bradycardia and tachycardia are relatively common in paediatrics. Their defining heart rates are listed in Table 6.2.

Bradycardia

Bradycardia may be due to hypoxia, acidosis and respiratory or circulatory failure, or it may be a pre-terminal event prior to cardiorespiratory arrest.

Table 6.2: Bradycardia and tachycardia heart rates (beats min⁻¹)

Age	Bradycardia	Tachycardia
< 1 year	< 80*	> 180
> 1 year	< 60	> 160

*although 80 min⁻¹ is defining rate for bradycardia in an infant chest compressions are not indicated until the heart rate is < 60 min⁻¹.

A bradycardic child with signs of decompensation or a child with a rapidly dropping heart rate associated with poor systemic perfusion requires immediate oxygenation (airway opening, 100% oxygen administration and positive pressure ventilation as necessary). If the heart rate remains < 60 min⁻¹ (all ages) and the child is unconscious with decompensated circulatory failure, chest compressions must also be started. The cause of the bradycardia must be sought and treatment directed at the underlying cause.

By far the commonest causes of bradycardia in infants and children are hypoxia and vagal stimulation. Less commonly, hypothermia and hypoglycaemia can slow conduction through cardiac tissues and result in bradycardia. Infants and children with a history of heart surgery are at increased risk damage to the AV node or other parts of the conduction system.

Atropine is indicated when increased vagal tone is the cause of the bradycardia (e.g. induced by tracheal intubation or suctioning). Otherwise adrenaline is the medication of choice but only once oxygenation has been restored and the HR remains < 60 min⁻¹ with circulatory failure. Very occasionally, in a child with congenital heart disease, the bradycardia is due to complete heart block, and emergency cardiac pacing is required. Pacing is not indicated in children with bradycardia secondary to hypoxic/ischaemic myocardial insult or respiratory failure.

Tachycardia

An elevated heart rate is frequently the normal physiological response to anxiety, pain or pyrexia. This is sinus tachycardia (ST) and is managed by treating the primary cause.

Other causes of ST include:

- respiratory conditions; early hypoxia, hypercarbia, obstructed airway and pneumothorax

- circulatory conditions; hypovolaemia, cardiac failure, anaphylaxis or sepsis, pulmonary hypertension

- miscellaneous causes; drugs, seizures.

The other cause of tachycardia is an arrhythmia, either supraventricular tachycardia (SVT) or ventricular tachycardia (VT).

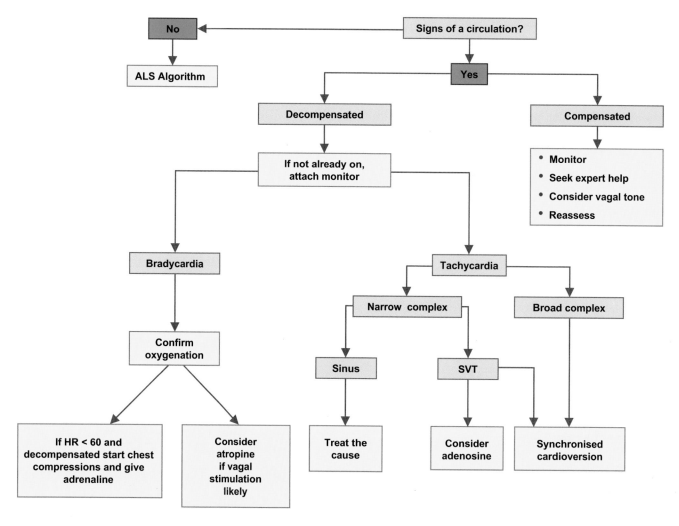

Figure 6.3 Managing the child with a cardiac arrhythmia

Of these, SVT is far more common in children. The priority of management is to establish whether the child is stable, or if they are displaying signs of circulatory decompensation. If the child is in a compensated state, expert help should be sought for definitive management.

The child who has decompensated circulatory failure requires chemical or electrical cardioversion whilst their ABCDE is continually assessed and appropriately supported.

4. Width of QRS complexes

In children with a tachycardia the most important thing to establish is whether this is ST or an abnormal rhythm (tachyarrhythmia). The history and clinical examination are key in determining this. The ECG features and width of the QRS complexes can also be helpful but it is always the child's clinical status that determines the urgency of management, regardless of the type of arrhythmia.

Narrow QRS complex tachycardia

Both ST (Figure 6.4) and SVT (Figure 6.5) have narrow QRS complexes, making it potentially difficult to differentiate

between them. The clinical and ECG differences that help to make this distinction are listed in Table 6.3.

Broad QRS complex tachycardia

In children, broad complex tachycardia is uncommon and usually due to an SVT. However, if uncertain, carefully consider VT (Figure 6.6) as this has more immediately serious consequences if inadequately treated (i.e. it can deteriorate to VF or pVT).

VT is usually found in a child who has underlying cardiac disease.

VT is broad complex, regular rhythm. The p waves are either absent or unrelated to the QRS complexes (Figure 6.6). It can present with or without a pulse; pVT is managed in the same manner as VF (i.e. with CPR and urgent defibrillation).

The management of VT with a pulse involves urgent expert consultation, as it has the potential to rapidly deteriorate to pVT or VF. The ongoing management of these children may involve electrical cardioversion or chemical

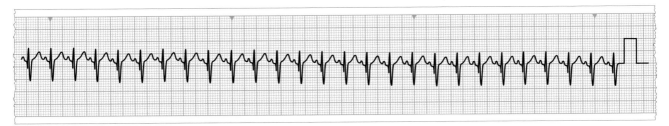

Figure 6.4 Sinus tachycardia rhythm strip

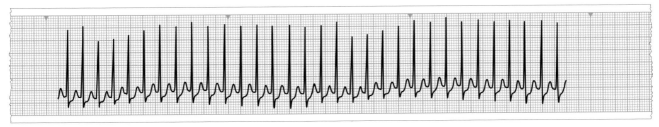

Figure 6.5 Supraventricular tachycardia rhythm strip

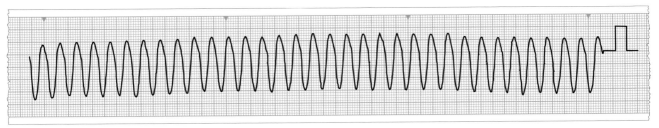

Figure 6.6 Ventricular tachycardia rhythm strip

cardioversion (usually with amiodarone). An anaesthetist or paediatric intensivist should be contacted in addition to a cardiologist as amiodarone can cause hypotension and may result in rapid circulatory decompensation and if electrical cardioversion is required anaesthesia may be necessary.

Supraventricular tachycardia

SVT is the most common primary cardiac arrhythmia observed in children. It is a paroxysmal, regular rhythm with narrow QRS complexes, caused by a re-entry mechanism through an accessory pathway or the atrioventricular conduction system. A heart rate of > 220 min⁻¹ in infants or > 180 min⁻¹ in children older than one year is highly suggestive of SVT. The other features that help to differentiate SVT from ST are listed in Table 6.3.

Management of SVT

Once a diagnosis of SVT is made, the child's clinical status will determine the management. As described previously, a child with compensated circulatory status should be referred for expert help. Treatment may include vagal manoeuvres, adenosine or cardioversion.

Vagal manoeuvres

In infants and small children, this can be performed by soaking a flannel in ice cold water, and then placing it briefly over their face. In cooperative children, a Valsalva manoeuvre can be induced by asking the child to blow through a drinking straw. A variation on this is to blow

Table 6.3 Clinical and ECG differences between ST and SVT		
	ST	**SVT**
History	Clues (e.g. pyrexia, fluid or blood loss)	Non specific Previous arrhythmia
Heart rate (beats min⁻¹)	Infant < 220 min⁻¹ Child < 180 min⁻¹	Infant > 220 min⁻¹ Child > 180 min⁻¹
P wave	Present and normal (N.B. not clearly seen at heart rates > 200 min⁻¹)	Absent or abnormal
Beat-to-beat variability (R – R)	Yes – can be altered with stimulation	None
Onset and end	Gradual	Abrupt

through the outlet of a syringe in an effort to expel the plunger.

Adenosine

If intravascular access is already established in a conscious, compensated child with SVT, chemical cardioversion with adenosine may be possible. Adenosine should be given rapidly via a vein as close to the heart as possible, as it is metabolised by red blood cells as soon as it enters the bloodstream.

A rapid bolus of 0.1 mg kg^{-1} should be followed with a flush of 2–5 mL 0.9% saline. If this dose is ineffective, it can be doubled (i.e. 0.2 mg kg^{-1}). The maximum dosages are 6 mg for the first attempt and 12 mg for the second. Caution: adenosine can precipitate severe bronchospasm. It causes unpleasant feelings of impending doom in the child and should ideally only be given under the guidance of a paediatric cardiologist.

Adenosine should be used with caution in heart transplant recipients and asthmatics.

Cardioversion

The procedure for undertaking synchronised electrical cardioversion is described in Chapter 7. It is the procedure of choice for decompensated children with SVT, particularly if they are unconscious. A general anaesthetic or deep sedation will be required if the child is conscious. The first shock should be delivered at the energy level of 1 J kg^{-1}, and the second (if required) at 2 J kg^{-1}. If the SVT fails to convert after a second shock, amiodarone maybe recommended before further shocks are delivered. This should ideally be under the guidance of a paediatric cardiologist or paediatric intensivist.

Summary learning

- **Life-threatening cardiac arrhythmias are more frequently the result, rather than the cause, of acute illness.**
- **The child's clinical status dictates management priorities – treat the patient not the monitor.**
- **The cause of the arrhythmia should be sought and treated.**

My key take-home messages from this chapter

Further reading

Brierley J, Carcillo JA, Choong K et al. Clinical practice parameters for hemodynamic support of pediatric and neonatal septic shock: 2007 update from the American College of Critical Care Medicine. Crit Care Med 2009; 37:666-688.

Carcillo JA, Davis AL et al Role of early fluid resuscitation in pediatric septic shock. JAMA. 1991; 266:1242-1 245.

Carpenter TC, Stenmark KR. High-dose epinephrine is not superior to standard dose epinephrine in pediatric inhospital cardiopul monary arrest. Pediatrics. 1997; 99:403-408.

de Oliveira CF, de Oliveira DS, Gottschald AF, et al. ACCM/PALS haemodynamic support guidelines for paediatric septic shock: an outcomes comparison with and without monitoring central venous oxygen saturation. Intensive Care Med 2008; 34:1065-75.

Dauchot P, Gravenstein JS. Effects on atropine on the electrocardiogram in different age groups. Clin Pharmacol Ther 1971; 12:274-280.

Ditchey RV, Lindenfels JA. Potential adverse effects of volume loading on perfusion of vitals organs during closed-chest resuscitation. Circulation. 1984; 69:181-185.

Goetting MG, Paradis NA. High-dose of epinephrine improves outcome from pediatric cardiac arrest. Ann Emerg Med.1991; 20:22-26.

Graf W, Brutocao D et al. Admission glucose level as a predictor of survival and neurological outcome in pediatric submersion victims. Ann Neurol. 1991; 30:473-477.

Losek JD. Hypoglycaemia and the ABC's (sugar) of pediatric resuscitation. Ann Emerg Med 2000; 35:43-46.

Olasveengen TM, Sunde K, Brunborg C, Thowsen J, Steen PA, Wik L.Intravenous drug administration during out-of-hospital cardiac arrest: a randomized trial. J Am Med Assoc 2009;302:2222–9.

Michaud LJ, Rivara LP et al. Elevated initial blood glucose levels and poor outcome following severe brain injuries in children. J Trauma 1991; 31:1356-1 362.

Patterson MD, Boenning DA, Klein BL et al. . the use of high-dose epinephrine for patients with out-of-hospital cardiopulmonary arrest refractory to prehospital interventions. Pediatr Emerg Care 2005;21:227-37.

Perondi MB, Reis AG, Paiva EF, Nadkarni VM, Berg RA. A comparison og high-dose and standard-dose epinephrine in children with cardiac arrest. N Eng J Med 2004;350:1722-30.

Srinivasan V, Spinella PC, Drott HR, Roth CL, Helfaer MA, Nadkarni V. Association of timing, duration and intensity of hyperglycemia with intensive care unit mortality in critically ill children. Pediatr Crit Care Med 2004;5:329-36.

Stiell IG, Wells GA, Field B, et al. Advanced cardiac life support in out-ofhospital cardiac arrest. N Engl J Med 2004;351:647–56.

Tenebein M. Continuous naloxone infusion for opiate poisoning in infancy. J Pediatr. 1988; 105:645-648, 1988.

Defibrillation and cardioversion

Contents

- **Definition of defibrillation**
- **Types of defibrillators**
- **Sequence of actions for defibrillation and cardioversion**
- **Defibrillation safety**

Learning outcomes

To enable you to:

- **Describe the indications for defibrillation and cardioversion**
- **Understand how to deliver safely an electrical shock using either a manual or automated external defibrillator (AED)**
- **Discuss how factors influencing the likelihood of successful defibrillation/cardioversion**

Incidence of shockable arrhythmias

Although the initial rhythm in a paediatric cardiorespiratory arrest is far more likely to be asystole or pulseless electrical activity (PEA) than ventricular fibrillation (VF) or pulseless ventricular tachycardia (pVT), a shockable rhythm is present in up to 27% of paediatric in-hospital arrests at some point during the resuscitation. When a shockable rhythm is present, the likelihood of a successful outcome is critically dependent on rapid, safe defibrillation.

A defibrillator can also be used in the management of a child with circulatory compromise due to VT with a pulse or supraventricular tachycardia (SVT) (Chapter 6). In these situations, the machine is used to perform synchronised DC (direct current) cardioversion, which is also described in this chapter.

Defibrillation

Defibrillation is the generic term used to describe the procedure of passing an electrical current across the myocardium with the intention of inducing global myocardial depolarisation and restoring organised spontaneous electrical activity. This electrical current may be delivered asynchronously when there is no cardiac output (in VF or pVT), or it may be synchronised with the R wave when there is an output (in SVT or VT with a pulse), the latter being called cardioversion.

The energy dosage should cause minimal myocardial injury. The electrical current delivered to the heart depends on the selected energy (in joules) and the resistance to current flow (thoracic impedance). If the impedance is high, the energy requirement will be increased.

EPALS

Factors determining thoracic impedance

The factors that potentially affect thoracic impedance and therefore the energy required include:

- defibrillator pads/paddles size

- interface between pads/paddles and the child's skin

- positioning of the pads/paddles on the chest wall

- chest wall thickness and obesity.

Types of defibrillators

Defibrillators are either automatic (i.e. automated external defibrillators (AEDs) or manually operated. They may be capable of delivering either monophasic or biphasic shocks. AEDs are pre-set for all parameters including the energy dose.

Manual defibrillators capable of delivering the full range of energy requirements for newborns through to adults must be available within all healthcare facilities caring for children at risk of cardiorespiratory arrest. Some manual defibrillators are capable of measuring depth and rate of chest compressions giving feedback about the quality of CPR being given.

In children requiring cardioversion (e.g. a child with circulatory failure from SVT) a manual defibrillator should be used.

Monophasic defibrillators

Monophasic defibrillators are no longer manufactured but may remain in use. They deliver a unipolar (one way) current.

Biphasic defibrillators

There are various types of biphasic waveform but there is no data to support one being superior to another. There is however, good evidence that biphasic defibrillators are more effective than monophasic ones. A biphasic defibrillator delivers a current that flows in a positive direction, and then in reverse for a specified duration. First shock efficacy for long-lasting VF/pVT is better with biphasic than monophasic waveforms. Biphasic waves also appear to cause less post-shock cardiac dysfunction.

Paddles or pads?

Manual defibrillation is now more commonly performed using self-adhesive pads (i.e. 'hands free' defibrillation) rather than using manual defibrillator paddles. Self-adhesive pads are safe, effective and generally preferable to defibrillator paddles. A major advantage of using self-adhesive pads is that they allow the rescuer to defibrillate from a safe distance, rather than having to lean across the patient; this is particularly important when access to the patient is restricted in a confined space. They deliver the shock more rapidly and with less interruption to CPR as the machine can be charged whilst chest compressions are in

progress. Some self adhesive pads have a sensor attached which measures rate and depth of chest compressions so that the rescuer can monitor the quality of CPR delivered.

> Rarely manual paddles are used; if they are, separate defibrillation gel pads first need to be applied to the child's chest wall to ensure good contact and reduce transthoracic impedance. These gel pads tend to fall off during chest compressions, often requiring repositioning before each defibrillation attempt. Additionally, they can lead to spurious asystole on ECG analysis as the gel becomes polarised and less effective as a conducting agent on repeated defibrillation attempts. This phenomenon is not encountered with the self-adhesive pads.
>
> If using the defibrillator paddles, the aim is to ensure the maximal contact with the chest wall. The largest available paddles should be selected but they must not come in to contact with each other. Generally, the standard (adult) size paddles are appropriate for use in children over 10 kg body weight. If the child is smaller than this, the infant paddles (approximately 4.5 cm diameter) should be used. If infant paddles are unavailable for use on a small child, then the standard paddles can be placed in an anteroposterior (front and back) position instead. When delivering the shock, firm pressure needs to be exerted onto the paddles by the rescuer.

Position of self-adhesive pads

Self-adhesive pads should be placed on the child's chest in a position that 'brackets' the heart to facilitate the flow of electrical current across it. The standard positioning is to place one pad just below the right clavicle to the right of the sternum and the other in the mid-axillary line on the left of the chest (Figure 7.1). Alternative pad position is anterior-posterior (Figure 7.2). Using this position, some defibrillators will provide feedback on the quality of chest compressions (rate, recoil and depth).

When using self-adhesive pads, it is essential to ensure that they do not touch each other. Selection of appropriate pads relating to the child's size/age may also be necessary, although this varies between manufacturers. The pads should be smoothed onto the child's chest ensuring that no air is trapped underneath as this will increase impedance and reduce the efficiency of the defibrillation shock. Although the pads are generally labelled right and left or have a diagram of their correct positioning on the chest, it does not matter if they have been reversed. Therefore if they have accidentally been placed the wrong way round they should be left in place and not repositioned. Repositioning results in time wasting and the self-adhesive pads may stick less effectively.

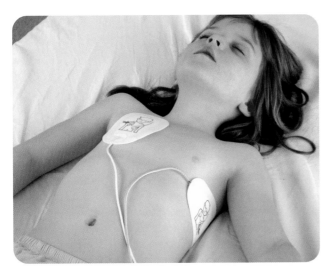

Figure 7.1 Self-adhesive defibrillation pads in position on a child

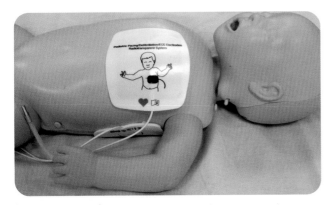

Figure 7.2 Self adhesive pads in the anterior-posterior position on an infant

Care must be taken when placing defibrillator pads/paddles on children who have an implantable cardioverter-defibrillator (ICD) or cardiac pacemaker, since the current delivered by an external defibrillator may travel along their wire/lead, resulting in burns where they are in contact with the myocardium. Manual defibrillation pads/paddles must be placed at least 12 cm from the pacemaker/ICD site; this may necessitate anteroposterior positioning in some children.

Defibrillation may increase the resistance at the contact point and the 'threshold' for pacing over a period of time. If resuscitation of these children is successful, the pacemaker threshold must be regularly checked for some months after the event.

Energy levels

Manual defibrillators

Manual defibrillators (Figure 7.3) have several advantages over AEDs and therefore must be readily available in all healthcare settings where children at risk of cardiorespiratory arrest may be cared for, even when AEDs are located nearby. The advantages include:

- ability to alter energy levels

- trained operators can diagnose arrhythmias and, when appropriate, deliver shocks more rapidly (with AEDs this diagnosis must await the results of the machine's rhythm analysis)

- additional facilities permit other treatments (e.g. synchronised cardioversion or external pacing).

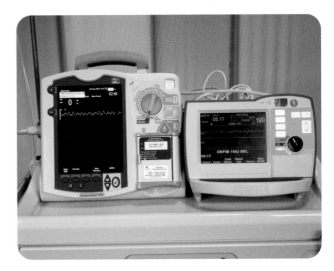

Figure 7.3 Manual defibrillators

When using a manual defibrillator an energy dose of 4 J per kg body weight (4 J kg^{-1}) should be used for all shocks, regardless of whether they are monophasic or biphasic waveforms. In a large child, the adult dosages should not be exceeded.

Automated external defibrillators

These machines are now widely available including through Public Access Defibrillation (PAD) schemes as fully or semi-automated devices (Figure 7.4). They are safe, reliable and sophisticated and are increasingly used by health professionals and lay rescuers.

If there is any likelihood of use in infants and small children check with the manufacturer that the machine is suitable. Machines with paediatric attenuation devices are preferable.

The AED will analyse the patient's ECG rhythm, determine whether a defibrillation shock is indicated and facilitate the delivery of a shock. In the semi-automated models, follow the AED prompts and press the relevant button.

Some of the models available to healthcare professionals have the facility for the operator to override the AED and deliver a shock independently of any prompting by the machine.

The main advantages of AEDs are that they recognise specific shockable rhythms and therefore a shock can be delivered by a lay-person. They are also relatively cheap and lightweight and have therefore replaced many manual defibrillators. Available AEDs have been tested extensively against libraries of adult ECG rhythms and in trials in adults and children. They are extremely accurate in rhythm recognition in both adults and children. The voice prompts from the AED must be followed to ensure safe, effective practice.

If a child > 25 kg (approximately eight years) requires defibrillation, standard adult AED energy levels can be used.

If a child of < 25 kg (or eight years) requires emergency defibrillation, and there is no manual defibrillator available, an AED can be used. The AED should ideally be equipped with a dose attenuator, which decreases the delivered energy to a lower, more appropriate dosage (generally 50–75 J). If such an AED is unavailable in an emergency situation, then a standard AED with adult energy levels may be used. The upper dose limit for safe defibrillation is unknown but higher doses than the previously recommended 4 J kg^{-1} have defibrillated children effectively and without significant adverse effects. Higher doses are acceptable because defibrillation is the only effective treatment for VF/pVT.

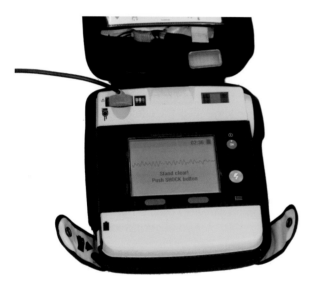

Figure 7.4 Automated external defibrillator (AED)

Infants have a much lower incidence of shockable rhythms and good quality CPR is the treatment priority. If an infant is in a shockable rhythm however and a manual machine is not available, use of an AED (preferably with attenuator) may be considered.

Minimal interruption to chest compression

Every time chest compression is interrupted, even for a brief period, coronary and cerebral perfusion pressure fall and several compressions are needed to return these pressures to their previous levels. Interruptions should therefore be minimised during the defibrillation sequence.

- If a shockable rhythm is still present the manual defibrillator should be charged whilst chest compressions are continued.

- Compressions should be resumed straight after the shock with no check of either the monitor or patient.

Safety issues when undertaking defibrillation

The safety of the rescuers as well as that of the child is paramount. The following factors must be considered:

Oxygen

All free-flowing oxygen delivery devices (O_2 masks or nasal cannulae) must be removed from the immediate area and placed at least one metre from the child. If the child is being ventilated via a tracheal tube, the ventilation bag or ventilator tubing can be left connected if it forms part of a closed circuit. If the circuit is disconnected for whatever reason, the devices must be placed at least one metre away from the child.

Dry surfaces

Any wet clothing should be removed from the immediate area. The surface the child is laid on and the child's chest should be wiped dry if necessary, before shock delivery.

Contact with patient

The person delivering the shock must ensure that neither they nor any other rescuers/relatives are in direct or indirect contact with the child during shock delivery.

There should be no contact between the pads and any metal objects (e.g. jewellery) or items such as transdermal medication or diathermy pads.

Operator instructions

Familiarity with the defibrillator being used increases safety and operator efficiency. Operators must also ensure that they issue clear instructions to the rest of the team/bystanders to facilitate safe practice throughout the procedure.

Sequence of actions for manual asynchronous defibrillation

If the ALS rescuer is first on scene the entire BLS sequence needs to be followed. If, however, the rescuer is part of a response team arriving to find BLS already ongoing they should perform a short simultaneous breathing and pulse check looking for signs of life. This should not need to take another full 10 seconds as the goal is to minimise time off the chest. The caveat is that the response team should feel confident that those performing BLS were certain of the diagnosis of cardiac arrest; if there is doubt then ALS providers may want to consider going back to the beginning of BLS sequence (this should be the rare scenario in a healthcare setting). This confirmation check is brief (approximately 5 seconds) as the first responder/s will have already completed a full 10 s check prior to commencing BLS. Furthermore, the team are about to embark on ALS where the rhythm analysis will be an additional tool for management.

Having confirmed cardiorespiratory arrest, CPR should be started (or restarted) while the person delivering the shock prepares as follows:

1. Confirm presence of shockable rhythm (VF/pVT) via self-adhesive/monitoring pads or ECG monitor during brief pause in chest compressions.

2. Resume chest compressions preferably using a sensor allowing CPR feedback.

3. The designated person selects the appropriate energy (4 J kg^{-1}) and presses the charge button.

4. While the defibrillator is charging warn all rescuers other than the individual performing the chest compressions to "stand clear", and remove any oxygen delivery device as appropriate.

5. Once the defibrillator is charged, tell the rescuer doing the chest compressions to "stand clear"; when clear and after confirming continued VF/pVT, give the shock.

6. Without reassessing the rhythm or feeling for a pulse, restart CPR starting with chest compressions.

7. Continue CPR for two minutes; the team leader prepares the team for the next pause in CPR (steps 3 and 4).

8. If VF/pVT persists deliver a second shock (as for steps 5 and 6).

Further management of shockable cardiac arrest rhythms is described in Chapter 8.

Considerations when using an AED

The AED pads are placed in the same position as manual defibrillators (Figure 7.1).

Sequence of actions for using an AED

The following guidance should be used for all AEDs, with or without a paediatric dose attenuating device:

1. Ensure safety of the child and rescuers/bystanders.

2. Start BLS. If more than one rescuer is available, one should summon help as appropriate, and then return to assist with BLS and attachment of the AED.

   If only one rescuer is available, they should perform one minute of CPR before going for help/collecting and attaching the AED (unless a cardiac cause is suspected).

3. Switch on the AED and attach self-adhesive pads. If more than one rescuer is present, BLS should be continued whilst the AED is attached.

4. Follow the AED prompts.

5. **Ensure no-one touches the child while the rhythm is being analysed.** This is extremely important as artefact from chest compressions given during analysis phase

may be interpreted by the AED as VF and the machine may charge and advise a shock.

6. If defibrillation is indicated:
   - ensure no-one touches the child
   - press the shock delivery button as directed
   - continue as directed by the AED prompts.

7. If no shock is indicated:
   - resume BLS immediately
   - continue as directed by the AED prompts.

8. Continue resuscitation until:
   - help arrives and takes over management
   - the child starts to show 'signs of life'
   - the rescuer becomes too exhausted to continue.

NB Do not switch off the AED whilst CPR is continued.

Testing the defibrillator

Defibrillators should be regularly tested as per manufacturer and local policies. All potential operators should familiarise themselves with the specific operating procedures of their available machines.

Considerations when undertaking synchronised DC cardioversion

Cardioversion is the timed delivery of an electrical shock from the defibrillator. It is a procedure that can be used in the treatment of symptomatic SVT or VT with a pulse. The delivery of the electric shock is synchronised with the R wave of the ECG to minimise the risk of inducing VF.

The application of the pads and the safety precautions are the same as for asynchronous defibrillation, but there are some additional considerations. These include:

- Sedation/anaesthesia needs to be administered (if the child is conscious) before synchronised cardioversion is performed.

- Synchronisation mode on the defibrillator must be activated and on some machines it may need to be re-selected if repeat shock(s) are required or if the machine is accidentally turned off between shocks.

- Increase the ECG gain to ensure the defibrillator identifies all the R waves on the child's ECG.

- Energy levels for synchronised cardioversion are lower than for asynchronous defibrillation. The initial dose is 1 J kg^{-1} although this may be increased to 2 J kg^{-1} if the arrhythmia persists.

- ECG electrodes in addition to pads are needed for some defibrillators to operate in the synchronised mode.

- Delay in shock delivery can occur between the operator depressing the delivery button and the actual shock being delivered. This is because the machine will only deliver the shock when it identifies an R wave. In practice it means that the operator must keep the shock delivery button depressed until this occurs.

Following cardioversion, some defibrillators may remain in the synchronised mode which is a potential risk; a defibrillator left in the synchronised mode will not be immediately ready to deliver a shock to treat a VF/ pVT cardiorespiratory arrest victim, therefore always leave the defibrillator in the non-synchronised mode.

Summary learning

- **For the patient in VF, early defibrillation is the only effective means of restoring a spontaneous circulation.**
- **When using a defibrillator, minimise interruptions in chest compressions.**
- **Use an AED if you are not confident in rhythm recognition or manual defibrillation.**

My key take-home messages from this chapter

Further reading

Atkinson E, Mikysa B et al. Specificity and sensitivity of automated external defibrillator rhythm analysis in infants and children. Ann Emerg Med 2003;42: 185-96.

Benson D, Jr., Smith W, Dunnigan A, Sterba R, Gallagher J. Mechanisms of regular wide QRS tachycardia in infants and children. Am J Cardiol 1982;49:1778-88.

Berg RA, Chapman FW et al. Attenuated adult biphasic shocks compared with weight-based monophasic shocks in a swine model of prolonged pediatric ventricular fibrillation. Resuscitation 2004; 61: 189-197.

Berg RA, Samson RA et al. Better outcome after pediatric defibrillation dosage than adult dosage in a swine model of pediatric ventricular fibrillation. J Am Coll Cardiol 2005;45: 786-9.

Clark CB, Zhang Y et al. Pediatric transthoracic defibrillation: biphasic versus monophasic waveforms in an experimental model. Resuscitation 2001;51: 159-63.

Edelson DP, Abella BS, Kramer-Johansen J, et al. Effects of compression depth and pre-shock pauses predict defibrillation failure during cardiac arrest. Resuscitation 2006;71:137-45.

Eftestol T, Sunde K, Steen PA. Effects of interrupting precordial compressions on the calculated probability of defibrillation success during out-of-hospital cardiac arrest. Circulation 2002;105:2270-3.

Faddy SC, Powell J et al. Biphasic and monophasic shocks for transthoracic defibrillation: A meta analysis of randomised controlled trials. Resuscitation 2003;8: 9-16.

Jorgenson D, Morgan C, Snyder D et al. Energy attenuator for pediatric application of an automated external defibrillator. Crit Care Med 2002;30:S145-7.

Meaney P, Nadkarni V et al. Effect of defibrillation dose during in-hospital pediatric cardiac arrest. Pediatrics 2011;127(1):e16-23.

Rodriguez-Nunez A, Lopez-Herce J. Shockable rhythms and defibrillation during in-hospital pediatric cardiac arrest. Resuscitation 2014;85:387-91.

Rossano JQ, Schiff L, Kenney MA, Atkins DL. Survival is not correlated with defibrillation dosing in pediatric out-of-hospital ventricular fibrillation. Circulation 2003;108: IV-320-321.

Seeram N, Wren C. Supraventricular tachycardia in infants: response to initial treatment. Arch Dis Child 1990;65:127-9.

Samson R, Berg R et al. Use of automated external defibrillators for children: an update. An advisory statement from the Pediatric Advanced Life Support Task Force, International Liaison Committee on Resuscitation. Resuscitation 2003;57: 237-43.

Schneider T, Martens PR et al. Multicenter, randomized, controlled trial of 150-J biphasic shocks compared with 200- to 360-J monophasic shocks in the resuscitation of out-of-hospital cardiac arrest victims. Circulation 2000;102: 1780-1787.

Tibbals J, Carter B et al. External and internal biphasic direct current shock doses for pediatric VF and pulseless VT. Pediatric Crit Care Med 2011;12:14-20.

Management of cardiorespiratory arrest

Contents

- **Resuscitation process**
- **In-hospital cardiorespiratory arrest**
- **Non-shockable rhythms**
- **Shockable rhythms**
- **Ongoing resuscitation**
- **Reversible causes of cardiorespiratory arrest**

Learning outcomes

To enable you to:

- **Plan for effective management of the resuscitation team**
- **Describe the importance of the team huddle**
- **Manage resuscitation until experienced help arrives**
- **Manage non-shockable cardiac arrest rhythms**
- **Manage shockable cardiac arrest rhythms**
- **Understand the importance of high quality cardiopulmonary resuscitation**
- **Identify the potentially reversible causes of cardiorespiratory arrest**
- **Consider when to stop resuscitation attempts**

Resuscitation process

The division between basic life support (BLS) and advanced life support (ALS) is somewhat artificial. Resuscitation is a continuous process, and the elements of effective BLS must be continued until return of a spontaneous circulation (ROSC), even when experienced help arrives (i.e. the EMS or clinical emergency team) and appropriate equipment can be used to facilitate delivery of advanced techniques. It is important that the on-call resuscitation team prepare for this event at changeover of staff and team huddles (Chapter 14).

All clinical staff within a healthcare facility should be able to:

- immediately recognise cardiorespiratory arrest
- start appropriate resuscitation (BLS with available adjuncts)
- summon the clinical emergency team using the standard telephone number (2222 in-hospital) and/or EMS (via national 999 or 112 system)

The exact sequence of actions will be dependent on several factors including:

- location of event (clinical or non-clinical area)
- number of first responders

EPALS

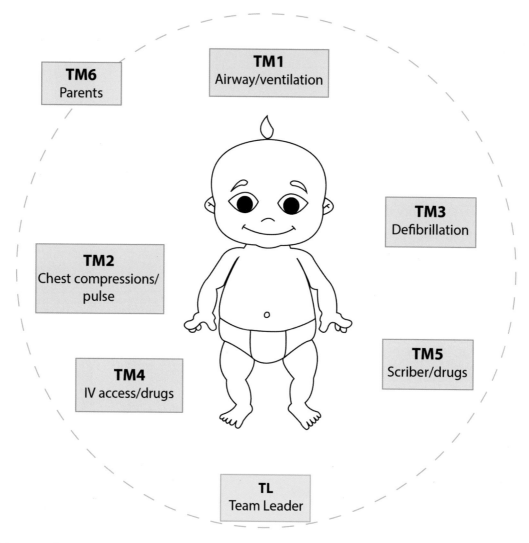

Figure 8.1 Diagram of team member organisation

- skills of first responders
- availability of resuscitation equipment
- local policies.

Location of event

Clinical area

If the child is seriously ill on a ward, it is likely that they will have been deteriorating over a period of time. Many wards now employ an 'early warning scoring system' based on physiological parameters (e.g. paediatric early warning score (PEWS)), which is designed to identify seriously ill children before they become decompensated; experienced staff are alerted and can initiate appropriate management strategies to try and prevent cardiorespiratory arrest occurring.

When a child does suffer a cardiorespiratory arrest in a clinical area staff should be able to promptly initiate BLS and put out a 2222 call to summon the clinical emergency/cardiac arrest team. Appropriate resuscitation equipment and trained staff should be readily available.

Non-clinical area

There may be occasions when a child suffers a cardiorespiratory arrest in a non-clinical area (e.g. corridors, car park, play area). In these areas, there may not be readily available equipment or trained staff, and these children may have a more prolonged period of BLS before help arrives.

The guidance in the first section of this chapter is primarily aimed at healthcare professionals who may be initial responders in a clinical emergency situation and have rapid access to resuscitation equipment. The guidance in the second section of this chapter is primarily aimed at the team providing experienced help including guidance for the team leader.

Number of first responders

A single rescuer must not leave the collapsed child, but should start appropriate resuscitation (e.g. BLS or BLS with BMV) and ensure that further help is summoned.

Within a clinical area, there are usually more staff nearby who can be alerted, either by the first responder shouting for help and/or using an emergency call button system. As soon as a second rescuer arrives, they should be sent to summon further assistance in line with local policy (i.e. activate the clinical emergency team; in hospitals this will be via a 2222 call). On their return (or the arrival of other staff) simultaneous interventions can be undertaken, according to the skills of the available staff.

Skills of first responders

Healthcare providers should be able to recognise cardiorespiratory arrest, shout for help and start resuscitation to the level to which they have been trained. The decay in resuscitation skills after training is well documented with skills retention probably lasting about 3 months. Recent studies indicate that short targeted refresher training for staff looking after the sicker patients at the bedside may be beneficial, so called 'just in time' training.

Staff will have been trained to different levels according to local policies; some may only undertake BLS, whilst others would be expected to undertake additional techniques to manage airway, breathing and circulation. First responders should only undertake the skills they have been trained to perform; their initial priority in paediatric cardiorespiratory arrest should be to ensure effective ventilation and oxygenation with good quality BLS. As more experienced help arrives, other interventions can be undertaken.

Availability of resuscitation equipment

All clinical areas where children are likely to be cared for should be equipped with resuscitation equipment to help with the management of a clinical emergency. The staff in each area should have responsibility for maintenance and regular checking of this clinical emergency equipment, as this will facilitate their familiarity with it. Standardised resuscitation equipment hospital-wide enables the clinical emergency team to know exactly what equipment is readily available to them when called to deal with a child in any area. Equipment capable of delivering CPR feedback for rescuers will improve the quality of CPR given and is advocated.

Quality standards

Healthcare organisations have an obligation to provide a high quality resuscitation service, and to ensure that staff are trained and updated regularly and with appropriate frequency to a level of proficiency appropriate to each individual's expected role. The Resuscitation Council (UK) *Quality standards for cardiopulmonary resuscitation practice and training* provide further detailed information.

Hospitals should also have policies regarding the composition of, and calling criteria for, their clinical emergency teams. In some centres, there might be more than one emergency team (dictated by the geographical layout or the clinical specialties of the hospital) or there may be different types of team (e.g. a cardiac arrest team and a medical emergency team). Staff must be aware of their local systems and trained to act accordingly. Operational issues should be audited. Continuous measurement of compliance with processes, and patient outcomes at a national and local level provides information on the impact of changes in

practice, identifies areas for improvement, and also enables comparison in outcomes between different organisations.

Cardiac arrest teams should meet at the beginning of each shift to introduce themselves to each other, discuss each team member's skills and assign roles. These 'huddles' will improve teamwork, particularly communication. Cardiac arrest teams will also operate more efficiently if their skills can be practised (and their effectiveness measured) by undertaking 'mock' emergency calls. This includes consideration of team organisation at a resuscitation event (Figure 8.1).

In-hospital cardiorespiratory arrest sequence

The initial management of a collapsed child is summarised in Figure 8.2.

Safety

The approach described in Chapter 3 should be followed to ensure firstly the safety of the rescuers and then that of the child. Whilst the risk of contracting infection is low, personal protective measures should be used as soon as practicable (e.g. gloves, aprons, eye protection, face masks). In situations where the child may have a severe infection (e.g. open TB, Swine flu or SARS) rescuers must be equipped with full protective measures. In areas where such children may be treated, this equipment should be immediately available.

Stimulate

The approach described in Chapter 3 should be followed to establish the responsiveness of an unconscious child.

Responsive child

If the child responds (i.e. they demonstrate 'signs of life'), the child should be assessed using an ABCDE approach. Appropriate interventions should be initiated and further relevant assistance summoned.

Unresponsive child

If the child is unresponsive (i.e. they do not demonstrate 'signs of life'), start BLS immediately whilst simultaneously shouting for more assistance.

Shout for help

The single rescuer must not leave the child but shout loudly for help and start BLS, using basic airway adjuncts and BMV if they are immediately available and activating a bedside emergency call button system if this is available.

If there is a second rescuer available they should be sent to summon more assistance, and return to help with the resuscitation attempt.

If resuscitation equipment is nearby, they should bring this to the bedside, but this must not delay calling the clinical emergency team.

Airway

The airway should be opened as described in Chapter 3. If suction is available, it may be necessary to use this to clear any secretions in the upper airway before proceeding to ventilation.

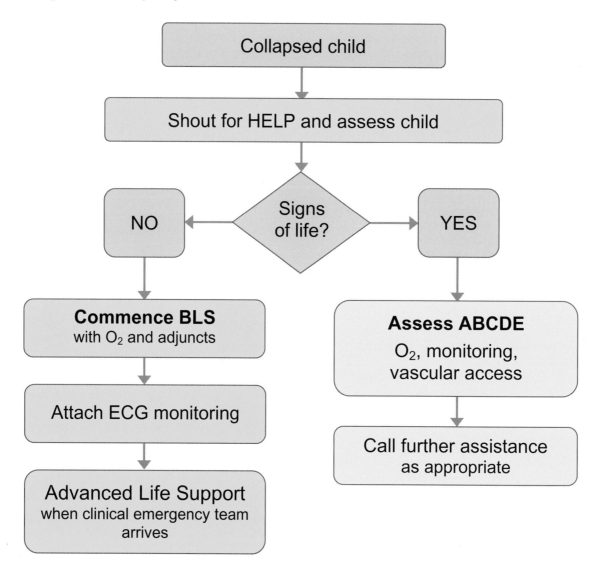

Figure 8.2 Initial resuscitation management

Breathing

If the child is not breathing, or only gasping ineffectively, initial rescue breaths should be delivered by the most appropriate method available (e.g. expired air rescue breaths with a barrier device or self-inflating bag-mask device with supplemental oxygen).

If there are two rescuers available and at least one is trained in the use of BMV, the rescuer managing the airway and delivering the rescue breaths should be positioned behind the child's head. A second rescuer should be positioned at the side of the child to perform chest compressions if indicated. As soon as resuscitation equipment is available, the emphasis is on ensuring that effective CPR is enhanced by BMV with supplemental oxygen.

Circulation

Assessment

If a child, who is not breathing adequately, does not respond quickly to rescue breaths, they are unlikely to have an adequate spontaneous circulation.

However, in the hospital setting, it is appropriate for a rescuer to take no more than 10 s to try and determine the presence of a central pulse whilst simultaneously observing for 'signs of life'.

If an adequate pulse (i.e. > 60 min^{-1}) is DEFINITELY felt, but breathing is absent or inadequate, the child's airway must be maintained and rescue breathing continued at a rate of 12–20 min^{-1}.

If the child's pulse is absent or inadequate (i.e. < 60 min^{-1}), or there is any doubt and there are no other 'signs of life', effective chest compressions must be started. Ventilations and compressions are then delivered in 15:2 ratio until monitoring is attached.

Rhythm recognition

Establish the child's cardiac rhythm by attaching an ECG monitor or defibrillator (preferably with a CPR feedback sensor). The priority is deciding whether the cardiac rhythm is shockable or non shockable, in order to determine the ongoing management of the cardiorespiratory arrest. If an AED is used, it will guide the rescuers through the sequence of actions. However, in paediatric areas of a hospital, an ECG monitor, usually a manual defibrillator, is commonly available and therefore the clinical emergency

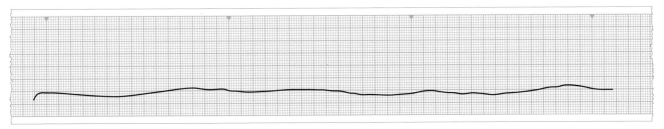

Figure 8.3 Asystole

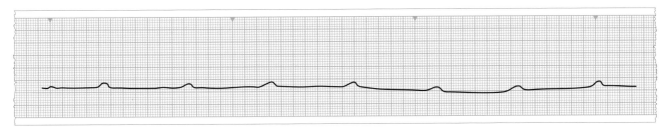

Figure 8.4 P-wave asystole

team members must be able to rapidly identify whether they are dealing with a child in a shockable or non-shockable rhythm. Briefly pause chest compressions to allow for rhythm recognition on the monitor.

Shockable or non-shockable cardiac rhythms

In children, the most common initial cardiorespiratory arrest rhythms are non-shockable (i.e. profound bradycardia, asystole or pulseless electrical activity (PEA)).

The shockable cardiorespiratory arrest rhythms (i.e. ventricular fibrillation (VF) and pulseless ventricular tachycardia (pVT)) are less common. When these occur, it is often in a child with underlying cardiac disease.

The management of shockable and non-shockable cardiorespiratory arrest is outlined below.

Non-shockable rhythms (asystole and PEA)

Asystole

This rhythm is characterised by the total absence of effective electrical and mechanical activity in the heart (Figure 8.3).

It can be simulated by artefact (e.g. detached ECG leads/electrodes) so it is important to quickly check the equipment. In asystole, there is no ventricular function, but occasionally there is some atrial activity, which may be seen on the ECG as P waves (Figure 8.4). It is often preceded by severe bradycardia. The most common cause of bradycardia in a child is hypoxia but hypotension, hypothermia or hypoglycaemia can depress normal cardiac activity and slow conduction through cardiac tissues.

Pulseless electrical activity (PEA)

This rhythm is defined as organised cardiac electrical activity in the absence of a palpable central pulse. Some of

these children may have some myocardial contraction, but it is too weak and ineffective to produce a detectable pulse or blood pressure. The ECG rhythm displayed is often a slow, broad complex one, although any variation of regular QRS complexes may be seen.

All the cardiac arrest rhythms may be due to an underlying reversible condition (see below); identify and treat all reversible causes listed within the paediatric advanced life support algorithm (Figure 8.5).

Management of asystole and PEA

- **Perform continuous CPR:**

  o Continue to ventilate with high-concentration oxygen.

  o If ventilating with bag-mask use a ratio of 15 chest compressions to 2 ventilations.

  o Use a compression rate of 100–120 min^{-1}. Depth approximately 4 cm in an infant, and 5 cm in a child.

  o If the patient is intubated, chest compressions can be continuous as long as this does not interfere with satisfactory ventilation.

  o Once the child's trachea has been intubated and compressions are uninterrupted use a ventilation rate of approximately 10–12 min^{-1}. Once there is return of ROSC, the ventilation rate should be 12–20 per min^{-1}. Measure end-tidal CO_2 to monitor ventilation and ensure correct tracheal tube placement.

- **Give adrenaline:**

  o If vascular access has been established, give adrenaline 10 mcg kg^{-1} (0.1 mL kg^{-1} of 1 in 10,000 solution) as quickly as possible.

  o If there is no circulatory access, obtain intraosseous (IO) access.

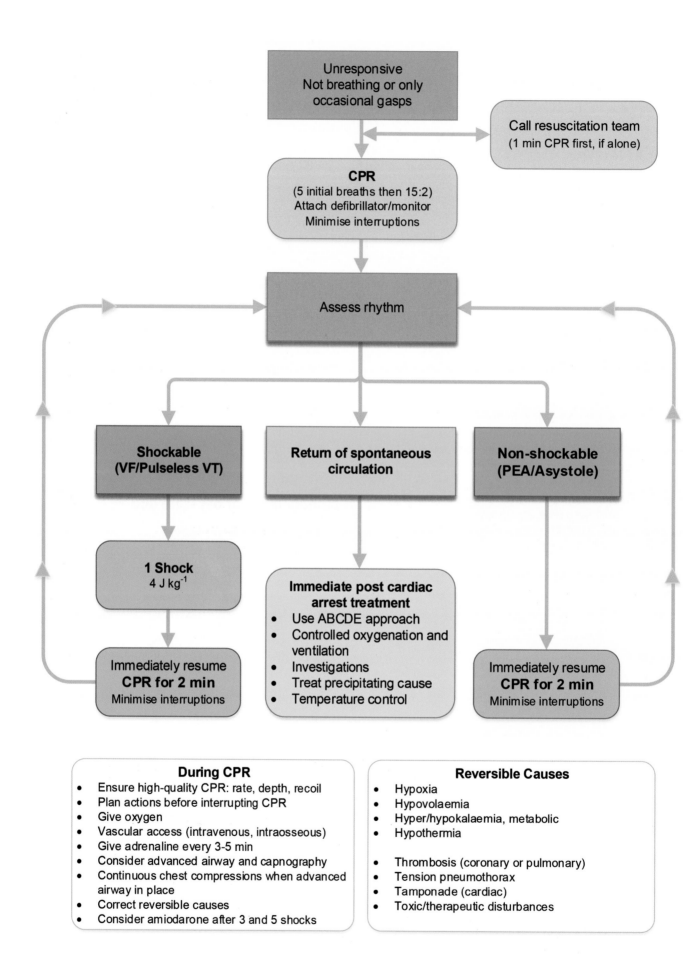

Figure 8.5 Paediatric advanced life support algorithm G2015

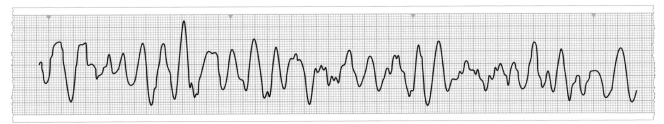

Figure 8.6 Coarse ventricular fibrillation

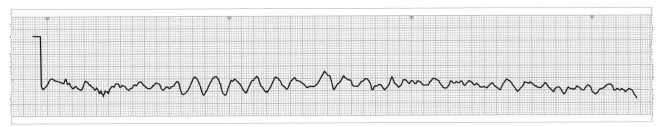

Figure 8.7 Fine ventricular fibrillation

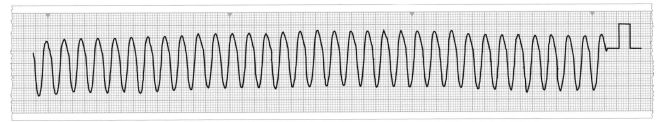

Figure 8.8 Ventricular tachycardia

- **Continue CPR, only pausing briefly every 2 min to check for rhythm change**

  o Give adrenaline 10 mcg kg^{-1} every 3–5 min, (i.e. every other loop), while continuing to maintain effective chest compressions and ventilation without interruption.

  o The aim is to maximise chest compression time and the chest compression fraction (CCF) should exceed 80%.

  o Good quality CPR is maximised if a feedback device is used.

- **Consider and correct reversible causes:**
  (4Hs and 4Ts)

- **If, during the rhythm check, organised electrical activity is seen on the monitor, check for 'signs of life' and a central pulse:**

  o If a pulse > 60 min^{-1} and/or 'signs of life' are present, start post-resuscitation care.

  o If there is no pulse, or you are unsure, and there are no 'signs of life' (i.e. PEA) continue with 'non-shockable' algorithm.

If the cardiac rhythm changes to ventricular fibrillation (VF) or pulseless ventricular tachycardia (pVT), the team must change their management to follow the shockable side of the paediatric advanced life support algorithm (Figure 8.5).

Shockable rhythms (VF and pVT)

Ventricular fibrillation

This rhythm shows rapid, chaotic, irregular waves of varying frequency and amplitude. VF is sometimes classified as 'coarse or fine' depending on the amplitude (height) of the complexes (Figures 8.6 and 8.7). When there is doubt as to whether a rhythm is fine VF or asystole, the team should not deliver a defibrillation shock but should continue with CPR. It is unlikely that fine VF will be successfully shocked into a perfusing rhythm, but continuing good quality CPR may increase the frequency and amplitude of the VF and improve the chances of successful defibrillation (i.e. to produce a perfusing rhythm). If the cardiac rhythm is clearly VF, defibrillation should be performed without delay.

Pulseless ventricular tachycardia (pVT)

This rhythm is a broad complex tachycardia (Figure 8.8). It is rare in children and is managed in the same way as VF (i.e. defibrillation).

Management of VF/pVT

- Continue CPR with BMV and supplemental O$_2$ until a defibrillator is available. The sequence below relates in particular to clinical areas using a manual defibrillator.

  - **Defibrillate the heart:**

    o Charge the defibrillator while another rescuer continues chest compressions.

    o Once the defibrillator is charged, pause the chest compressions, quickly ensure that all rescuers are clear of the patient and then deliver the shock. This should be planned before stopping compressions.

- o Give 1 shock of 4 J kg⁻¹ if using a manual defibrillator.
- • **Resume CPR:**
  - o Without reassessing the rhythm or feeling for a pulse, resume CPR immediately, starting with chest compression.
  - o The aim is to maximise chest compression time and the chest compression fraction (CCF) should exceed 80%.
  - o Good quality CPR is maximised if a feedback device is used.
  - o Consider and correct reversible causes (4Hs and 4Ts).
- • **Continue CPR for 2 min, then pause briefly to check the monitor:**
  - o If still VF/pVT, give a second shock (with same energy level and strategy for delivery as the first shock).
  - • **Resume CPR:**
    - o Without reassessing the rhythm or feeling for a pulse, resume CPR immediately, starting with chest compression.
- • **Continue CPR for 2 min, then pause briefly to check the monitor:**
- • **If still VF/pVT, give a third shock** (with same energy level and strategy for delivery as the previous shock).
  - • **Resume CPR:**
    - o Without reassessing the rhythm or feeling for a pulse, resume CPR immediately, starting with chest compression.
    - o Give adrenaline 10 mcg kg⁻¹ and amiodarone 5 mg kg⁻¹ after the third shock, once chest compressions have resumed.
    - o Repeat adrenaline every alternate cycle (i.e. every 3–5 min) until ROSC.
    - o Repeat amiodarone 5 mg kg⁻¹ one further time, after the fifth shock if still in a shockable rhythm.
- • Continue giving shocks every 2 min, continuing compressions during charging of the defibrillator and minimising the breaks in chest compression as much as possible.
  - o **After each 2 min of uninterrupted CPR, pause briefly to assess the rhythm: If still VF/pVT:**
    - ■ Continue CPR with the shockable (VF/pVT) sequence.
  - o **If asystole:**
    - ■ Continue CPR and switch to the non-shockable (asystole or PEA) sequence as above.

- o **If organised electrical activity is seen**, check for signs of life and a pulse:
  - ■ If there is ROSC, continue post-resuscitation care.
  - ■ If there is no pulse (or a pulse rate of < 60 min⁻¹), and there are no other signs of life, continue CPR and continue as for the non-shockable sequence above.
- • If defibrillation was successful but VF/pVT recurs, resume the CPR sequence and defibrillate. Give an amiodarone bolus (unless two doses have already been given) and start a continuous infusion of the drug.

Important note

Chest compressions should be interrupted only briefly for defibrillation and ventilations and chest compression fraction should be maintained above 80%. Chest compression delivery is tiring for providers and the team leader should repeatedly assess and feedback on quality of the compressions. Studies show that visual assessment of depth of compressions is inaccurate therefore where possible feedback devices should be utilised. When correct guideline depth and rate are achieved the chances of survival are markedly improved.

Rationale for sequence of actions on shockable side of algorithm

- • The interval between stopping chest compressions and delivering a shock must be minimal (< 10 s); longer interruptions to chest compressions reduce the likelihood of a shock restoring a perfusing rhythm.

- • Chest compressions are resumed immediately after a shock without reassessing the rhythm or feeling for a pulse because, even if the defibrillation attempt is successful in restoring a rhythm, it is unlikely that the heart will immediately pump effectively. Even if a perfusing rhythm has been restored, giving chest compressions does not increase the chance of VF recurring.

If an organised rhythm is observed during a 2 min cycle of CPR, **do not interrupt chest compressions to palpate a pulse, unless the patient shows signs of life** demonstrating return of spontaneous circulation (ROSC).

If there is any doubt about the presence of a pulse in a patient who has an organised cardiac rhythm compatible with cardiac output, but no other signs of life, resume CPR for a further 2 min.

Ongoing resuscitation

Outcome in all resuscitation attempts is dependent on teamwork with good quality chest compressions and ventilation (plus defibrillation when indicated for shockable arrhythmias). Performing chest compressions is tiring so the emergency team members should pre-plan sharing the work by alternating nominated team members every two minutes, ensuring seamless changeover and minimising chest compression interruptions. As soon as the airway is secured with a tracheal tube, chest compressions should be performed continuously unless this compromises delivery of adequate tidal volumes.

Airway and ventilation

The vast majority of children can be adequately ventilated with BMV in the initial stages of resuscitation; it is often better to continue with this until ROSC rather than attempt tracheal intubation and temporarily interrupt chest compressions and oxygenation during laryngoscopy. However, once the expertise is available, tracheal intubation provides the most reliable airway and will be essential in the post-resuscitation management of a child who has suffered cardiorespiratory arrest.

If laryngoscopy is to be performed during CPR, it should be attempted without interruption of chest compressions, although there may need to be a brief pause as the tracheal tube is passed through the vocal cords.

Following tracheal intubation and confirmation of the correct tube position, it should be secured and then chest compressions can be delivered continuously without a pause for ventilation. If possible end-tidal carbon dioxide levels should be continuously monitored as they provide feedback on the effectiveness of ongoing CPR. **Breaths should be delivered at a rate of 10–12 min⁻¹ (i.e. one breath every 5 or 6 s), this is much slower than is usually performed.**

History and reversible causes

Obtaining relevant information about the child's underlying medical condition and any pre-disposing events can be useful in determining likely causes of, and potential outcome from, the cardiorespiratory arrest.

The 4 Hs

1. **Hypoxia**
2. **Hypovolaemia**
3. **Hypo/hyperkalaemia/metabolic**
4. **Hypothermia**

The 4 Ts

1. **Tension pneumothorax**
2. **Tamponade (cardiac)**
3. **Toxins/therapeutic disturbance**
4. **Thrombosis (coronary or pulmonary)**

Any possible causes (or aggravating factors) that have specific treatment must be considered during all cardiorespiratory arrests. The most likely of these can be recalled by the mnemonic '4 Hs and 4 Ts':

Hypoxia

This is a frequent cause of paediatric cardiorespiratory arrest. The risks of it occurring, or persisting, during resuscitation should be minimised by ensuring effective ventilation with 100% oxygen. It is essential to ensure that there is adequate, bilateral chest movement.

Hypovolaemia

Loss of circulating volume can often result in cardiorespiratory arrest. When a child shows signs of circulatory failure, controlled volume administration is indicated. Hypovolaemia may be due to many different causes (e.g. haemorrhage from trauma, diarrhoea and vomiting, anaphylaxis, severe sepsis) and these need to be identified and treated appropriately. If signs of circulatory failure are present, start rapid circulatory volume replacement with an initial bolus of 0.9% saline solution; volume and frequency of bolus is discussed in Chapter 5.

Hypo/hyperkalaemia, metabolic causes

Electrolyte and metabolic disorders may be suggested by the child's medical history and/or biochemical tests. Specific treatment should be given to correct these problems. An estimation of blood glucose level should be obtained early; both hypo and hyperglycaemia are common and associated with increased morbidity and mortality.

Hypothermia

Low body temperature may be an unlikely problem in hospitalised children, but it should always be considered, particularly in small or premature infants, or in children being managed in the emergency department. A low-reading thermometer should be used to record a core temperature when hypothermia is considered a possibility. If the child's temperature is > 34 °C they should not be actively rewarmed.

Tension pneumothorax

Signs of tension pneumothorax (e.g. decreased chest movement and air entry, hyper-resonance on the affected side, tracheal deviation away from the affected side) should be sought, particularly in children who have suffered trauma, following thoracic surgery or jugular or subclavian vein central line insertion. If a tension pneumothorax is thought to be present, rapid needle decompression is required, followed by chest drain insertion.

Tamponade (cardiac)

This is not a common cause of cardiorespiratory arrest in children, but may occur following cardiothoracic surgery, penetrating chest trauma or some viral illnesses. It can be difficult to diagnose as typical signs (e.g. distended neck veins and hypovolaemia) are often masked by the cardiorespiratory arrest. If there is a strong history, needle pericardiocentesis is indicated.

Toxins/therapeutic disturbance

In the absence of a confirmed history, accidental or deliberate poisoning with toxins (therapeutic or toxic substances (e.g. digoxin toxicity, tricylic antidepressant overdose)) may only be discovered after laboratory analysis. Appropriate antidotes should be administered as soon as possible when indicated and available, but frequently management of these children is based on measures to support their vital organs. Check the child's drug chart.

Thrombosis (coronary or pulmonary)

It is unusual for children to suffer from thromboembolic complications, but they can occur. If suspected, appropriate thrombolysis would be needed (e.g. Alteplase as per local guidelines).

Stopping resuscitation

Resuscitation efforts are less likely to be successful in achieving ROSC if there have been no signs of cardiac output, despite at least 30 min of continuous, good quality CPR in children. However, occasionally good quality survival has been reported for longer durations of CPR, so the circumstances of the cardiac arrest, the age and the presenting rhythm must all be taken into consideration when making the decision to stop resuscitation; CPR is more often successful in children > 1 year of age and in those presenting with VF or pVT.

It would be appropriate to prolong resuscitation attempts in children with the following conditions:

- hypothermia
- poisoning
- persistent VF/ pVT.

The resuscitation team may also consider that specific circumstances (e.g. awaiting arrival of family members) make it appropriate to maintain resuscitation efforts.

Presence of parents during resuscitation

The opportunity to be present during at least part of the resuscitation of their child should be offered to parents/carers. Evidence suggests that this aids with their grieving process (less anxiety and depression when assessed several months later).

The following points (which apply whether the parent is actually in the room beside their child, or elsewhere in the ward/department) should be considered:

- A specific member of staff should be delegated to remain with the parents throughout to offer empathetic, but realistic, support.

- If necessary, an appropriate interpreter must be present to facilitate accuracy of communication between parents and the resuscitation team leader.

- Physical contact with their child and the opportunity to say 'goodbye' (in unsuccessful resuscitation attempts) should be encouraged.

- The resuscitation team leader decides when to stop resuscitation efforts, and not the parents.

- A debriefing session for all staff involved should be arranged to offer support and reflect on practice.

- Appropriate referrals and counselling should be organised for the parents to ensure they receive adequate support.

Summary learning

- **The optimal management of in-hospital cardiorespiratory arrest is always based on the rapid initiation of effective ventilation, oxygenation and good quality chest compression.**

- **The paediatric advanced life support algorithm provides a framework for cardiopulmonary arrest management with an emphasis on providing good quality CPR with minimal interruptions in chest compression delivery.**

- **Asystole and PEA are non-shockable arrhythmias and their management is based on effective CPR, adrenaline administration and treatment of reversible causes.**

- **VF and pVT are shockable arrhythmias and their management is based on effective CPR, early defibrillation and treatment of reversible causes.**

- **The parents/carers should be supported and, ideally, be present during the resuscitation of their child.**

My key take-home messages from this chapter

Further reading

ILCOR 2015 worksheets on resuscitation
www.americanheart.org/presenter.jhtml?identifier=3060115
References to the basis for resuscitation including the presence of relatives
in the resuscitation room are available from this website.

Duncan HP, Frew E: Short-term health system costs of paediatric in-hospital
acute life-threatening events including cardiac arrest. Resuscitation
2009;80:529-534.

Edwards ED, Mason BW, Oliver A, Powell CV: Cohort study to test the
predictability of the melbourne criteria for activation of the medical
emergency team. Arch Dis Child 2010.

Eppich WJ, Brannen M, Hunt EA: Team training: Implications for emergency
and critical care pediatrics. Curr Opin Pediatr 2008;20:255-260.

Hanson CC, Randolph GD, Erickson JA, Mayer CM, et al. A reduction in cardiac
arrests and duration of clinical instability after implementation of a
paediatric rapid response system. Postgrad Med J 2010;86:314-318.

Nolan JP, Soar J, Zideman DA, Biarent D et al. European Resuscitation
Council Guidelines for Resuscitation 2010 Section 1. Executive summary.
Resuscitation. 2010;81:1219-76.

Thomas EJ, Williams AL, Reichman EF, Lasky RE, et al. Team training in the
neonatal resuscitation program for interns: Teamwork and quality of
resuscitations. Pediatrics 2010;125:539-546.

Tibballs J, Kinney S: Reduction of hospital mortality and of preventable
cardiac arrest and death on introduction of a pediatric medical emergency
team. Pediatr Crit Care Med 2009;10:306-312.

Topjian AA, Nadkarni VM, Berg RA: Cardiopulmonary resuscitation in
children. Curr Opin Crit Care 2009;15:203-208.

Van Voorhis KT, Willis TS: Implementing a pediatric rapid response system to
improve quality and patient safety. Pediatr Clin North Am 2009;56:919-933.

Weinstock P, Halamek LP: Teamwork during resuscitation. Pediatr Clin North
Am 2008;55:1011-1024, xi-xii.

Winberg H, Nilsson K, Aneman A: Paediatric rapid response systems: A
literature review. Acta Anaesthesiol Scand 2008;52:890-896.

EPALS

Post-resuscitation care, stabilisation and transfer

Contents

- Post cardiac arrest syndrome pathology and management
- Preventing secondary injury via ABCDE assessment and management
- Preparing for transfer/retrieval of children to other facilities for ongoing care

Learning outcomes

To enable you to:

- Understand the importance of post-resuscitation stabilisation and optimisation of organ function following cardiorespiratory arrest
- Describe the specific investigations and monitoring indicated
- Facilitate the safe transfer of the seriously ill child

Continued resuscitation

Cardiorespiratory arrest represents the most severe shock state during which delivery of oxygen and metabolic substrates to tissues is abruptly halted. Cardiopulmonary resuscitation (CPR) only partially reverses this process, achieving cardiac output and systemic oxygen delivery that is much less than normal. The aim is to restore oxygenation and perfusion to the vital organs as rapidly as possible to minimise the primary injury. For children who have had a cardiorespiratory arrest the initial step is restoration of spontaneous circulation (ROSC) but this is only the first step in the continuous process of resuscitation management. A significant percentage of resuscitated children ultimately die or survive with serious neurological sequelae so good post-resuscitation care is required to maintain organ perfusion and prevent secondary organ injury whenever possible.

Secondary organ damage includes:

- hypoxic-ischaemic brain injury
- ischaemic myocardial damage
- hypoxic pulmonary damage
- acute renal failure
- coagulopathy
- ischaemic hepatitis
- acute gastro-intestinal lesions.

The ABCDE approach must be followed in the immediate post-resuscitation phase as it focuses management priorities. However, the ongoing care of the child requires the expertise of many healthcare professionals and is best delivered in a paediatric intensive care (PICU) facility. This may require a specialist team to facilitate an optimal safe transfer.

EPALS

EUROPEAN PAEDIATRIC
ADVANCED LIFE SUPPORT

Stabilisation of airway and breathing

The aim of respiratory management is to maintain adequate oxygenation and ventilation, avoiding hypoxia, hyperoxia and hypo/hypercapnia, which may worsen the child's prognosis.

If the child (or infant) has been resuscitated using BMV a decision needs to be made whether he will need ongoing ventilation and placement of a tracheal tube. Factors that may affect this decision include:

- conscious level (AVPU) at level P or less means that there will be no protective airway reflexes

- requirement for the safe transfer to a PICU

- lung pathology resulting in a need for respiratory support.

BMV causes gastric distention which will impede ventilation and may cause vomiting. A gastric tube is usually required to deflate the stomach if it has become distended following BMV.

Children and infants who remain intubated and ventilated will need sedation and analgesia in most cases.

Following intubation, the most common post-resuscitation airway/breathing complications can be identified by considering the acronym DOPES (Table 9.1).

Table 9.1 Possible airway and breathing complications following tracheal intubation

D	Displacement of tracheal tube (e.g. oesophagus, right main stem bronchus)
O	Obstruction of artificial airway (accumulated secretions, kinking)
P	Pneumothorax (from excessive BMV pressure, rib fractures)
E	Equipment failure (e.g. disconnected oxygen supply)
S	Stomach distension (following expired air or bag-mask ventilation)

Vital signs, such as blood gases and SpO_2 must be monitored post-resuscitation.

SpO_2 should be monitored continuously with a pulse oximeter and blood gas analysis should be performed as soon as possible. Although 100% oxygen is used for resuscitation, prolonged administration of high oxygen concentrations can result in pulmonary and cerebral toxicity. Once the child is stable, inspired oxygen should be gradually reduced to achieve an SpO_2 of between 94–98%.

Exceptions are for children who have suffered smoke inhalation (carbon monoxide or cyanide poisoning) or have severe anaemia when a high FiO_2 should be maintained as dissolved O_2 helps in oxygen transport in these circumstances.

End-tidal CO_2 monitoring is essential. This will confirm the correct location of a tracheal tube, allow continuous CO_2 monitoring during transport and support the optimisation of ventilation to maintain normocapnia. A chest X-ray should be obtained to identify lung pathology, check for rib fractures (very rare in children) and confirm the correct tracheal and gastric tube positions (Figure 9.1).

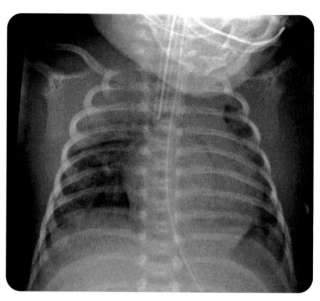

Figure 9.1 Chest X-ray showing tracheal tube at low position, causing right upper lobe collapse – this resolves when the tube is gently pulled back up the trachea.

If a resuscitated child has a tracheal tube in place and starts to make respiratory effort but remains unconscious, it is usually preferable to leave them intubated and ventilated (with appropriate sedation and analgesia) until after transfer and admission to PICU, since they can deteriorate rapidly, and reintubation during transfer is extremely hazardous.

Circulation

The aim of circulatory management is to ensure adequate organ perfusion and tissue oxygenation.

Haemodynamic function and cardiac rhythm are likely to be unstable in the immediate post-resuscitation phase but every effort should be made to try to optimise cardiac output and maintain blood pressure in the normal range. In addition to continuous ECG, SpO_2, end-tidal CO_2 and BP monitoring, vital organ perfusion should be assessed by recording urine output and peripheral perfusion (CRT and skin temperature) as a minimum. Ideally capillary refill time (CRT) should be < 2 s and the heart rate, blood pressure and respiratory rate should all be maintained within the age-appropriate range.

Systolic and mean BP are indirect measures of organ perfusion and can be obtained either non-invasively or continuously via an arterial line, (particularly useful for ventilated patients). Urine output should be > 1mL kg^{-1} h^{-1} in children. Assessment of central venous pressure (CVP), a measure of preload (i.e. the filling volume of the heart) may also be appropriate in some children but will require insertion of a central line. After fluid resuscitation palpation of the liver edge may also give an indication of fluid status (particularly in infants) and should normally be < 1 cm beyond the costal margin.

Assessment of the child's fluid balance and circulating volume must be considered. Resuscitation boluses of isotonic saline solutions, such as 0.9% saline or Hartmann's solution may be required to optimise circulating volume. Crystalloids can be safely used in the peri-resuscitation period but some patients may require blood or other colloids.

Maintenance fluids should be based on biochemistry evaluations and blood glucose should be measured. Glucose should be administered judiciously as required to avoid hypoglycaemia or hyperglycaemia as both conditions can have a deleterious effect on neurological outcome in critically unwell children. Careful monitoring is required. During the immediate post-resuscitation period, decisions about securing longer-term vascular access will be required (e.g. insertion of central venous cannulae to replace intraosseous access or additional lines to deliver specific medications).

Ongoing resuscitation of the child may necessitate inotrope infusions. These are preferably administered via dedicated central venous catheters. Having a central line with multiple lumens ensures that inotropes are not interrupted to deliver other medications and fluids, and avoids incompatibilities.

Commonly used inotropes include adrenaline and noradrenaline but consensus guidelines for specific conditions should be followed (e.g. sepsis guidelines for children).

Disability

The brain is highly vulnerable to hypoxia and ischaemia. It can be injured by direct trauma, infection, hyper/hypoglycaemia, hypocapnia, seizures or raised intracranial pressure. Secondary brain injury can be minimised by stabilising systemic blood pressure, treating seizures, normalising blood gases (taking particular care to avoid hypoxia) and correcting glucose and electrolyte abnormalities.

An assessment of neurological status should be performed early to obtain a post-resuscitation baseline, help identify neurological deficits and possibly help to predict prognosis.

Conscious level should be assessed with either the AVPU or Glasgow Coma Scale scoring systems. Pupil reactivity, posturing and focal signs should also be noted and regularly recorded.

Neuroprotective care post-ROSC aims to avoid secondary brain injury and should start from the first minutes after ROSC.

- **Cerebral perfusion:** immediately following ROSC, there may be a period of unstable cerebral blood flow. Cerebral perfusion is dependent on mean arterial pressure – hypotension or severe hypertension will compromise cerebral blood flow and may worsen any neurological injury. The aim is therefore to maintain the mean arterial pressure at, or slightly above, the child's normal level.

- **Seizure control:** the occurrence of seizures post-resuscitation is not uncommon and an isolated event does not appear to affect outcome. However, status epilepticus is associated with a poor outcome, and therefore control of seizure activity is essential to prevent increased cerebral metabolism and potential neurological injury. Commonly used treatments for seizure (e.g. benzodiazepines, phenytoin) can cause hypotension, and the BP and ECG needs to be closely monitored.

- **Ventilation:** studies suggest that ventilation to normocapnia is appropriate (4.5–6.0 kPa) as the response of the cerebral circulation to changes in CO_2 appears preserved. Low levels of CO_2 may therefore result in vasoconstriction and reduced cerebral blood flow and high levels of CO_2 to vasodilation and high cerebral blood flow; both of these may aggravate any brain swelling which occurs after cardiac arrest.

- **Temperature Control:** after ROSC strict control of temperature to avoid hyperthermia (>37.5°C) and severe hypothermia (<32°C) is mandatory. Hyperthermia post cardiorespiratory arrest is common in the first 48 h and is known to worsen brain injury with an increase in morbidity for every 1°C above 37°C; hence fever should be treated aggressively with antipyretics and active cooling. Initial trials of therapeutic hypothermia (TH) in adults following cardiorespiratory arrest showed improvement in survival and neurological outcome, however subsequent trials have failed to support these findings. Recent studies appear to show it is the avoidance of fever which may confer a better outcome rather than the application of TH per se in adults post cardiorespiratory arrest. A recently published large paediatric randomised controlled trial comparing mild TH (32–34°C) with therapeutic normothermia (36.8°C) post in-hospital cardiorespiratory arrest did not demonstrate any significant difference in survival or one year functional outcome between the two groups. There were no differences in complications between the two groups and it was concluded that TH appeared a safe therapy. The successfully resuscitated child with hypothermia and ROSC should not be immediately rewarmed actively unless the temperature is less than 32°C.

- **Blood glucose:** hypoglycaemia (< 3 mmol L^{-1}) and hyperglycaemia are associated with worse neurological outcome. Studies have not shown that tight control of blood glucose levels confers any benefit for paediatric patients and it carries the risk of inadvertent hypoglycaemia so it is not recommended. Glucose should be delivered as a continuous infusion rather than as boluses and blood glucose levels should be monitored frequently.

- **Maintenance fluids:** maintenance fluids should be started in children with choice of fluid directed by electrolyte and blood glucose measurements; usually 0.9% saline with or without 5 or 10% dextrose, or Hartmann's solution can be used. Maintenance requirements are best prescribed at 70–90% of normal values in critically unwell children.

- **Analgesia and sedation:** if children do not show adequate signs of awakening within the first 10 min after ROSC, mechanical ventilation and ongoing analgesia and sedation will be required. Adequate analgesia and sedation will reduce oxygen consumption, facilitate ventilation and prevent complications. The prevention and treatment of pain and the maintenance of an adequate level of sedation is therefore a priority. There are many sedatives, analgesics and muscle relaxants, but it is best to become familiar with the use of a small range, knowing their indications, beneficial actions and adverse effects. Although some of these drugs are used as continuous infusions in the PICU, outside the PICU bolus administration may be easier. Repeated reassessment is then required to ensure that the effect of bolus dose has not worn off. Never administer a neuromuscular relaxant without ensuring that the child is deeply sedated and will remain so. Sedation may not be necessary in profound coma and may interfere with neurological evaluation; always discuss such cases with the local PICU for guidance.

Exposure

Exposure and a full examination to detect any lesions (e.g. rashes, wounds) should be undertaken and may help in making the diagnosis, informing specific management of the child (e.g. the purpuric rash of meningococcaemia may prompt treatment with broad spectrum antibiotics if not already given). Care should be taken to respect the child's dignity and excessive hypothermia avoided especially in infants.

Other organs

Renal function should be monitored by measuring urine output, and the serum urea and creatinine levels. Insertion of a urinary catheter may be necessary. Treatment is directed towards maintaining an adequate circulating volume, which sustains renal perfusion. Hence diuretics are only indicated if decreased urine output persists after adequate fluid resuscitation. The gastrointestinal mucosa and liver can also be affected by hypoxia and ischaemia. Gastrointestinal mucosal injury can contribute to multi-organ failure, due to leakage of toxins and bacteria into the circulation. Treatment is aimed at maintaining adequate circulating volume and gut perfusion.

Further assessment

History

A comprehensive history is important to determine the cause of cardiorespiratory arrest, and plan ongoing management. This should include relevant details about the past medical history, previous health/ill health and medications, as well as precipitating events. Details about the initial management of the current event (e.g. delay in starting resuscitation) should also be sought, as these may influence ongoing management.

Investigations

The child's physiological parameters are likely to be deranged in the immediate post-resuscitation period; urgent haematological, biochemical, radiological and cardiological investigations may all be indicated (Table 9.2).

Table 9.2: Post-resuscitation investigations	
Investigation	**Rationale**
Arterial blood gas (plus lactate)	• Ensure adequate ventilation • Assess tissue perfusion
Biochemistry	• Assess renal function • Maintain normoglycaemia • Assess electrolyte balance (especially Na$^+$, K$^+$, Mg^{2+}, Ca$^+$) • Liver function tests to look for ischaemic injury
Full blood count Clotting screen Group and Save	• Assess haemoglobin level and exclude anaemia • Monitor infection markers (e.g. white cell count, CRP etc) • Identify underlying blood disorders • Assess any coagulopathy from sepsis or ischaemia • Allows for urgent crossmatch
Chest X-ray	• Establish position of tracheal tube, central venous lines, gastric tube (as appropriate) • Detect underlying pathology (primary respiratory or cardiac disease, aspiration) • Exclude pneumothorax/rib fractures • Establish heart size
Other investigations as indicated (e.g. head CT or pelvis X-rays, cardiac echography, 12-lead ECG, serum and urine toxicology)	

Blood gas interpretation

The ability to interpret a blood gas can give important information about the patient to help guide further management. The following is a simple guide to basic blood gas analysis.

The parameters commonly measured are: pH, PaO_2, $PaCO_2$, standard bicarbonate (SB), base excess (BE) and lactate. Directly measured values are: pH, $paCO_2$, paO_2, glucose and lactate. Calculated values are SB, BE and O_2 saturation (unless a Co-oximeter is used).

- **The pH** is a negative logarithm of hydrogen ion concentration in the blood (a decrease in pH from 7.0 to 6.0 indicates a ten-fold increase in concentration of H+ ions). It is a scale that measures the acid-base balance. Its normal range in the human body is **7.35 to 7.45.** Staying within this normal range is important for the body's enzymes and biological processes to work optimally.

- The body therefore regulates its **acid-base balance** tightly, by means of both the kidney and the respiratory systems. Acid is produced by most biological processes. This is initially buffered in the blood by a number of systems; the most important being the bicarbonate/carbonic acid system.

  o The kidneys can excrete excess acid in the urine and can also generate bicarbonate ions; these responses usually take hours.

  o Carbon dioxide partially dissolves in plasma forming carbonic acid. High carbon dioxide levels (hypercapnia, as in hypoventilation) result in an acid load and a fall in pH. Low carbon dioxide levels (hypocapnia, as in hyperventilation) can cause a rise in pH; these (ventilatory) responses usually take minutes.

Simple blood gas analysis

- STEP 1: Is the pH normal?

  If the pH is < 7.35 this is this called acidaemia

  If the pH is > 7.45 this is this called alkalaemia

- STEP 2: Is there a metabolic or respiratory abnormality or both?

  Metabolic acidosis is defined as
  SB ≤ 22 mmol/L

Metabolic alkalosis is defined as
SB > 26 mmol/L

Respiratory acidosis is defined as $paCO_2$ > 6 kPa (45 mmHg)

Respiratory alkalosis is defined as $paCO_2$ < 4.5 kPa (35 mmHg)

- STEP 3: Is the metabolic or respiratory abnormality compensated, partially compensated or uncompensated?

A respiratory or metabolic abnormality can exist with or without an acidaemia or alkalaemia. This is because the body will try and compensate for any abnormality and correct the pH.

Example 1: if there is a metabolic acidosis then the respiratory centre will be stimulated and the patient will hyperventilate causing the carbon dioxide level to fall resulting in a respiratory alkalosis. In this scenario the pH will initially be normal as the respiratory system compensates but eventually the compensatory mechanisms will fail and the pH will start to fall resulting in an acidaemia.

Example 2: a child with profound shock who is unconscious may be unable to mount a respiratory response to the metabolic acidosis and may present with a metabolic and respiratory acidosis with no compensation.

Blood gas interpretation			
pH	CO₂	HCO₃	Interpretation
<7.35	↑		Respiratory acidosis and acidaemia
<7.35		↓	Metabolic acidosis and acidaemia
>7.45	↓		Respiratory alkalosis and alkalaemia
>7.45		↑	Metabolic alkalosis and alkalaemia
<7.35	↑	↓	Combined acidosis and acidaemia
>7.45	↓	↑	Combined alkalosis and alkalaemia

Consequences of an abnormal blood gas

Once a blood gas has been interpreted, the causes of the abnormalities can be sought. Metabolic or respiratory acidosis with or without an acidaemia are the commonest abnormalities seen in the acutely unwell child. An alkalosis in acute illness may be due to poisonings (e.g. salicylate overdose).

- Causes of **respiratory acidosis** include for instance pneumonia, asthma, neuromuscular disorders and coma.

- Causes of **metabolic acidosis** include among others diarrhoea and vomiting, sepsis, heart failure, diabetic ketoacidosis and/or any form of shock (causing hypoperfusion and tissue hypoxia).

To help determine the cause of a metabolic acidosis various further tests can be performed such as chloride levels and anion gap but these are outside the scope of this discussion.

Measuring the pH of the blood gives information about the severity of the child's condition but it is also important as it in itself affects the circulation and oxygen delivery in different organs and tissues. Changes in pH affect the oxy-Hb dissociation curve. A rise in $paCO_2$ and drop in pH causes pulmonary vascular resistance to rise affecting blood flow to the lungs. The cerebral circulation is also affected by pH and $PaCO_2$: when the $PaCO_2$ rises and the pH drops the cerebral blood vessels dilate and cerebral blood flow increases – this may not be desirable in children who have cerebral oedema. When $PaCO_2$ drops and pH increases there is cerebral vasoconstriction which may potentiate any cerebral ischaemia.

Facilitating safe patient transfer

Following cardiorespiratory stabilisation, the child should be safely transferred to an appropriate (PICU) for definitive and ongoing medical support. The decision to transfer should be made only after discussion between senior members of the PICU team, the clinical emergency team leader and the child's primary team (if available for consultation). Other considerations pre-transfer are listed in Figure 9.2.

The transfer/retrieval team, whether in-hospital, or between hospitals, must be sufficiently experienced to be able to deliver any life-saving emergency interventions during the transfer period in any location (e.g. in an ambulance). The transfer team must be able to continue optimal clinical observations and perform all emergency interventions that may be necessary to manage a critically ill child during the transfer period in any location (e.g. in an ambulance). In the UK, a dedicated paediatric transfer/retrieval team will usually be involved. There are some circumstances however, such as intra-cranial bleeds and blocked VP shunts that require urgent neurosurgical intervention where rapid transfer by the most experienced available local team (most commonly the anaesthetic/emergency medicine/intensive care consultants) will be in the child's best interest.

- Stabilise the child (ongoing or recurrent cardiorespiratory arrest precludes transfer).

- Arrange the most appropriate mode of transport.

- Inform the paediatric consultant and any other specialty lead involved in the immediate care of the child (e.g. anaesthetist, surgeon, department nurse in charge, child protection lead if appropriate).

- Inform child's parents of transfer details and ensure they have appropriate means of transport to the PICU.

- A. Ensure a secure airway (aspirate any endotracheal tube secretions prior to transfer).

- B. Ensure appropriate settings on transport ventilator, adequate portable oxygen supplies for length of journey, and alternative means of ventilating the child (manual ventilation circuit that can be used either with or without oxygen supply). Deflate stomach with passage of a gastric tube.

- C. Ensure adequate intravenous access.

- D. Ensure adequate sedation and analgesia being delivered +/- muscle relaxant and that sufficient drugs are available for the journey. Reassess pupillary reaction and conscious level.

- E. Ensure heat loss during transfer is kept to a minimum (unless intentionally cooling the patient) with insulation blankets and warming devices.

- F. Fluids: Ensure maintenance fluids are running and blood glucose levels are monitored. Consider a urinary catheter prior to transfer. Monitor urine output. Transfer all medication/fluid infusions and monitoring to portable transport devices.

- Contact PICU to update them of child's clinical status and provide estimated time of arrival before departure.

- Prepare full and clear records of the event including all interventions (copies of notes, drug charts, X-rays is ideal).

- Just prior to moving the child run through the ABCDE assessment aloud with all team members involved. Request any suggestions or comments from the team and then confirm with all team members that they are in agreement to move the patient.

Figure 9.2 Pre-transfer considerations

Information required by the paediatric transport service

If inter-hospital transfer is required then a referral to a dedicated paediatric transport service may be required. Even if the transfer is time critical and the in-house team will be transferring the child then the paediatric transport service should still be contacted as they will assist in locating the nearest and most available bed and with emergency medical advice.

Certain information is required for this referral as detailed below:

- Childs details: (name, date of birth, gender, weight – actual or estimated).

- Referrers details: your name, position, attending consultant paediatrician and whether they have been informed of the transfer yet.

- Childs medical details: presenting complaint, past medical history including gestational age at birth, immunisation history, risk of contagious disease stratification and HPA involvement (recent travel, recent contagious contacts). Any child protection concerns.

- Details of any cardiorespiratory arrest: onset time of cardiorespiratory arrest, time of ROSC, location of arrest, special circumstances (i.e. submersion, hypothermia).

- Status currently: stable unstable; compensated decompensated.

- Treatment delivered so far: number of resuscitation cycles given and medications delivered before ROSC. Type and amount of fluid given, other medications given. Airway type; mode of ventilation; type of venous access or intraosseous access; neurological status and sedation muscle relaxant being delivered; body temperature and cooling or warming required; fluids being given, presence of anuria, suspicion of intra-abdominal or intra-thoracic mass.

- Investigation results: blood results, blood gases, any imaging performed.

Care and support of the child's relatives/main carers

The relatives of the child will require considerable ongoing support in the event of·both successful and unsuccessful resuscitation attempts. The early involvement of pastoral/counselling services should be considered.

There is evidence to suggest (in western societies) that by allowing parents to be present during their child's resuscitation witnessing the severity of the situation and the efforts made whatever the outcome can assist with the grieving process.

If parents wish to be present during the resuscitation, then a sufficiently experienced member of the resuscitation team should be allocated to support the parents and provide a commentary and explanation of the evolving events. The parents should always be offered the opportunity of leaving the room at any point. However, the allocated team member should continue to support the parents and provide updates on the status in the resuscitation.

Care of the rescuers/debriefing

It is important that all resuscitation events are audited (including the National Cardiac Arrest audit). Whether the resuscitation attempt was successful or not, healthcare providers should be supported and given constructive feedback on performance (Chapter 14).

Summary learning

- **ROSC following cardiopulmonary resuscitation is merely the first step in the continuous process of resuscitation management.**

- **The ongoing management of seriously ill children includes appropriate vital sign monitoring, supportive therapies based on continuous ABCDE assessment and safe transfer to a PICU facility.**

- **The prognosis for children following cardiorespiratory arrest depends on many factors, including the quality of post-resuscitation care.**

- **The ability to predict the neurological outcome of children following cardioplumonary resuscitation remains limited.**

My key take-home messages from this chapter

Further reading

Brierley J, Carcillo JA, Choong K et al. Clinical practice parameters for hemodynamic support of pediatric and neonatal septic shock: 2007 update from the American College of Critical Care Medicine. Critical Care Medicine 2009 37(2):666-88.

Macrae D, Grieve R, Allen E et al. A Randomized Trial of Hyperglycemic Control in Pediatric Intensive Care. New England Journal of Medicine. 2014. 370; 107-118.

Moler FW, Silverstein FS, Holubkov R et al. Therapeutic Hypothermia after Out-of-Hospital Cardiac Arrest in Children. New England Journal of Medicine. 2015. 372. 1898-1908.

Moler FW, Silverstein FS, Holubkov R et al. Therapeutic Hypothermia after In-Hospital Cardiac Arrest in Children. New England Journal of Medicine 2017;376:318-329.

Paediatric illnesses

Contents

- **Laryngotracheitis**
- **Epiglotitis**
- **Bacterial tracheitis**
- **Bronchiolitis**
- **Anaphylaxis**
- **Asthma**
- **Cardiac problems**
- **Sepsis**
- **Coma**
- **Seizures and metabolic**
- **Electrolyte disorders**

Learning outcomes

To enable you to:

- **Identify common paediatric illnesses**
- **Modify the ABCDE approach in certain paediatric illnesses**
- **Describe the management of some electrolyte disturbances encountered in critically ill children**

In childhood, cardiorespiratory arrest is mainly secondary to injury or illness and its outcome is poor; therefore strategies to recognise and manage diseases early may prevent progression to organ failure and cardiorespiratory arrest. Initially, recognition of respiratory and/or circulatory failure are more important than making a precise diagnosis of the disease. However, in certain circumstances, knowledge of specific disease processes may help to appropriately manage the disease and improve the outcome.

Illnesses affecting the airway

Laryngotracheitis (croup)

Croup is defined as an acute clinical syndrome of inspiratory stridor, barking cough, hoarseness, and variable degrees of respiratory distress. Acute viral laryngotracheobronchitis (viral croup) is the most common form of croup and accounts for over 95% of laryngotracheal infections.

Parainfluenza viruses are the most common pathogens but other respiratory viruses (e.g. respiratory syncytial virus (RSV) and adenoviruses) produce a similar clinical picture.

The majority of children with croup are managed at home, whilst those in mild to moderate respiratory distress may need admission and supportive treatment.

Steroids may be used to reduce laryngeal oedema. An oral steroid, dexamethasone, shows clear benefit even in mild cases of croup in reducing airway oedema; improvement in symptoms is seen within 2 to 3 h. One to two doses may be given. A few children may require intubation owing to a combination of exhaustion and respiratory failure.

- **Airway** – This is at risk of marked swelling of the larynx and trachea which can lead to partial or complete obstruction of the airway, if the oedema progresses. If the child is conscious and breathing let him adopt the preferred position, as manipulation or agitation will increase respiratory effort and obstruction. However, if the infant/child is decompensating, open the airway, give 100% oxygen and start bag-mask ventilation (BMV) if required. Advanced airway management is needed in only a few severe cases. It may be a challenge and inexperienced interference may worsen the situation. Help should be called in the form of an experienced team. A narrower tracheal tube than would normally be expected may be required.

- **Breathing** – Respiratory rate and work of breathing increase with progressive airway obstruction but may start to fall when the obstruction is more severe and decompensated respiratory failure occurs. Respiratory monitoring should be established and 100% oxygen given. Nebulised adrenaline can be given to reduce airway oedema (3–5mL of 1:1,000 adrenaline) for children with severe respiratory distress. Improvement is seen in minutes but wears off after 1 to 2 h after which there may be rebound oedema. Nebulised steroids such as budesonide can be given with nebulised adrenaline if child is vomiting and unable to take dexamethsone. Nebulised budesonide is equivalent to but not superior to dexamethasone in effectiveness. Rarely BMV will be needed in preparation for an advanced airway (in this case the two-person technique may be required). Respiratory failure is due to upper airway obstruction and will improve when the airway is adequately managed.

- **Circulation** – This is normal until decompensated respiratory failure develops.

- **Disability** – Exhaustion is an ominous sign, indicating decompensated respiratory failure.

Epiglottitis

This is an intense swelling of the epiglottis and surrounding tissues caused almost exclusively by Haemophilus influenzae type B. It is predominantly seen in children aged one to six years. It is now very uncommon owing to the availability of the Hib vaccination for children in the UK.

Typically, the child suddenly develops a high fever and is lethargic, pale and toxic. He is usually sitting immobile with his mouth open and chin raised. There may be excessive drooling owing to an inability to swallow saliva as it is painful to do so.

- **Airway** – Swelling of the epiglottis leads to severe obstruction of the upper airway causing stridor. Complete obstruction is fatal and can occur if the condition is untreated or if the child becomes distressed (e.g. by attempting to examine his throat, forcing him to lie down or performing other frightening manoeuvres such as inserting an intravenous cannula or taking a lateral X-ray of the neck). The child should be left with his parents, and under close observation, while arrangements are made for an experienced team to secure his airway by tracheal intubation under controlled conditions. Once the airway has been secured, normalisation of breathing is the rule. Thereafter, with intravenous antibiotics, the prognosis is excellent as the underlying infection usually responds quickly to treatment.

    If cardiorespiratory arrest occurs, the child should be ventilated by BMV (with pressure limiting valve being overridden if necessary) and this should be continued until the child is intubated or a surgical airway obtained.

- **Breathing** – There is an increased respiratory rate and effort, a muffled or hoarse voice, respiratory stridor and absent or minimal cough. Respiratory failure is due to the upper airway obstruction.

- **Circulation** – This is normal until decompensated respiratory failure develops. Inappropriate management can lead to sudden cardiorespiratory arrest because of complete airway obstruction.

- **Disability** – Tiredness and decreasing level of consciousness are worrying signs of decompensated respiratory failure. Exhaustion is a pre-terminal state.

- **Exposure** – The child may be dribbling saliva, looking flushed, 'toxic' and unwell. There is no specific rash to see.

Bacterial Tracheitis

This is a bacterial infection of the trachea resulting in the formation of mucopurulent exudates (that can form 'membranes') which may acutely obstruct the upper airway, this can be life-threatening. It is now more prevalent than epiglottitis. It is most common in children between the ages of three and eight years and should be considered in any child with signs of upper airway obstruction not responding to croup management. Presentation can be acute or subacute with barking cough, stridor, and fever.

- **Airway**: Signs of upper airway obstruction are present with stridor and barking cough. Don't agitate the child and call early for senior help. If the child acutely deteriorates it is usually because of movement of the membrane and BMV should be effective. Many children will need intubation and a tracheal tube half to one size smaller should be used to prevent further trauma to the inflamed subglottic area. Frequent suctioning and high humidity of inspired air and oxygen will be needed to prevent tube obstruction.

- **Breathing**: There is tachypnoea and increased respiratory effort, respiratory stridor and cough. Respiratory failure is due to the upper airway obstruction.

- **Circulation**: – This is normal until decompensated respiratory failure develops. Inappropriate management can lead to sudden cardiorespiratory arrest because of complete airway obstruction.

- **Disease specific management:** Once the airway has been stabilised intravenous access should be obtained for intravenous antibiotics. Broad spectrum antibiotics effective against staphylococcus and streptococcus species are indicated. Frequent airway toilet will be required for children who have been intubated.

Illnesses affecting breathing

Bronchiolitis

Bronchiolitis is a common, serious respiratory infection of infancy caused by RSV in 75% of cases; the remainder are due to parainfluenza, influenza and adenoviruses. It occurs mainly in the winter and is the reason for 1–2% of all infant admissions to hospital. 90% of patients are aged one to nine months and it is uncommon after one year. A subset of infants are at higher risk of developing more severe disease: infants less than three months old; infants with congenital heart disease; ex-premature infants; infants with chronic lung disease and infants with immunodeficiency. As there is no specific treatment for bronchiolitis, its management is supportive.

- **Airway** – Nasal obstruction from secretions can occur. Gentle suction of the nose will remove secretions if nasal obstruction impairs air entry.

- **Breathing** – The inflammatory process causes oedema of the small airways and copious secretions, which can lead to hypoxia and hypercapnia; a ventilation-perfusion mismatch occurs. Apnoea and exhaustion can also occur. The ventilation-perfusion mismatch may necessitate mechanical ventilation, although many children may be managed by continuous positive airway pressure (CPAP) through a well-fitted interface (e.g. nasal prongs or facial mask). Non-invasive ventilation is the first choice of management for respiratory failure in infants with bronchiolitis in many centres. Mechanical ventilation is required in 3% of hospitalised infants overall but 15–25% of high risk infants may need assisted ventilation. This may be due to recurrent apnoea, exhaustion or hypercapnia and hypoxia owing to small airway obstruction.

- **Circulation** – This is normal until decompensated respiratory failure occurs.

- **Disability** – Tiredness, confusion and agitation reflect failing respiratory compensation. Decreasing level of

consciousness is an ominous sign and exhaustion is a pre-teminal event.

Asthma

The UK continues to have the highest prevalence of childhood asthma in Europe, with significant related morbidity and mortality when compared to our European counterparts. 1.1 million children in the UK are currently receiving treatment for asthma (1 in 11 children) and 40 children die each year in the UK from asthma. The majority of asthma-related deaths occur before hospital admission. Cardiac arrest can be caused by hypoxia, tension pneumothorax, dynamic hyperinflation or secondary arrhythmias (caused by drugs or electrolyte disorders).

Expiratory wheezing is found as a sign of lower airway obstruction. There is no correlation between the severity of wheezing and the degree of obstruction. There are different causes of wheezing that present alternative diagnoses to exclude (e.g. anaphylaxis, foreign body aspiration, subglottic mass, pneumonia, bronchiolitis).

- **Airway:** the airway is normally open but can become obstructed when consciousness decreases.

- **Breathing:** respiratory monitoring should be established and supplemental oxygen administered as required. As long as there is compensated respiratory failure, avoid distressing the child, being aware that agitation may also be a sign of ongoing hypoxaemia. The absence of wheezing may indicate a critical obstruction, whereas increased wheezing may indicate a positive response to bronchodilation.

The severity of the asthma attack can be evaluated by monitoring oxygen saturations and the child's clinical status and response to treatment. If there are clinical signs of decompensation or exhaustion with decreasing consciousness an arterial blood gas is indicated (normal $PaCO_2$ values despite tachypnoea are indicative of worsening respiratory failure with values > 6.5 k Pa associated with life-threatening asthma). In the case of decompensated respiratory failure it might become necessary to support ventilation. Indications for intubation in asthma include: severe hypoxia, cardiac or respiratory arrest, rapid deterioration in conscious level. Intubation should be performed, whenever possible, by skilled personnel. BMV might be difficult because of increased airway resistance; be careful to avoid gastric inflation.

- **Circulation:** might be normal, but equally dehydration or obstructive shock (caused by pneumothorax or dynamic hyperinflation) can occur. If dehydration is suspected, a fluid bolus should be given, as hypovolaemia will further compromise circulation in patients with dynamic hyperinflation.

- **Management**

The early management of asthma is detailed in Figure 10.1.

- o **Nebulised/inhaled beta-2 agonists:** are first line agents for an acute asthma attack and should be administered as early as possible.

Recognition of asthma

These clinical features increase the probability of a diagnosis of asthma:
- More than one of the following: wheeze, cough, difficulty breathing and chest tightness. The risk is increased if these symptoms are recurrent, worse at night or in the early morning, occur during or after exercise or trigger dependent (e.g. with exposure to pets, cold, humidity, heightened emotions or occurring independent of upper respiratory tract infections)
- Personal history of atopic disorder
- Family history of atopic disorder and/or asthma
- Widespread wheeze heard on auscultation
- History of improvement in symptoms or lung function in response to adequate therapy.

Acute asthma in children under 2 years

The assessment of acute asthma in early childhood can be difficult
- Intermittent wheezing attacks are usually due to viral infection and the response to asthma medication is inconsistent
- Prematurity and low birth weight are risk factors for recurrent wheezing
- The differential diagnosis of symptoms includes: – aspiration pneumonitis – pneumonia – bronchiolitis – tracheomalacia – complications of underlying conditions such as congenital anomalies and cystic fibrosis.

Classification of severity of acute presentation

Moderate	Acute Severe	Life-threatening
• Normal mental state • Ability to talk in sentences or vocalise as normal • Some accessory muscle use • PEF ≥ 50% of best or predicted • O$_2$ saturations > 92% in air • Moderate tachycardia HR ≤ 125 min^{-1} (> 5 years) HR ≤ 140 min^{-1} (2–5 years) • RR ≤ 30 min^{-1} (> 5 years) • RR ≤ 40 min^{-1} (2–5 years)	• Agitated, distressed • Can't complete sentences in one breath • Moderate to marked accessory muscle use • PEF 33–50% of best or predicted • O$_2$ saturations < 92% in air • HR > 125 min^{-1} (> 5 years) • HR > 140 min^{-1} (2–5 years) • RR > 30 min^{-1} (> 5 years) • RR > 40 min^{-1} (2–5 years)	• Confused, drowsy, exhausted • Unable to talk • Maximal accessory muscle use (poor respiratory effort is pre-terminal) • Marked tachycardia (sudden fall in HR is pre-terminal) • PEF < 33% of best or predicted • O$_2$ saturations < 92% in air • Silent chest • Cyanosis • Hypotension

Management

Moderate	Acute Severe	Life-threatening
• Continuous O$_2$ saturation monitoring • High flow O$_2$ via face mask titrated to achieve O$_2$ saturations 94–98% • β2 agonist 2–10 puffs via pMDI + spacer +/-facemask, repeat dose every 20 min reviewing effect; no improvement in 1 h treat as acute severe. • Ipratropium bromide given early via pMDI + spacer +/- facemask, particularly if poorly responsive to β2 agonist • Oral steroids: 20 mg prednisolone for children aged 2 to 5 years; 30 to 40 mg for children > 5 years	• Continuous O$_2$ saturation monitoring • High flow O$_2$ via face mask titrated to achieve O$_2$ saturations 94–98% • β2 agonist nebulised (salbutamol 2.5–5mg) every 20 min with Ipratropium bromide (250mcg) for first 2 h; review frequently. • Consider adding magnesium sulphate 150mg to each β2 and Ipratropium bromide nebuliser in the first hour in children with a short duration of acute asthma presenting with oxygen saturations of < 92% • Oral steroids: 20 mg prednisolone for children aged 2 to 5 years; 30 to 40 mg for children > 5 years • Consider aminophylline if child unresponsive to maximal doses of bronchodilators and steroids • Consider ABG if poor response to early treatment	Continuous O$_2$ saturation monitoring • High flow O$_2$ via face mask titrated to achieve O$_2$ saturations 94–98% • Refer to PICU • β2 agonist nebulised (salbutamol 2.5–5mg) every 20 min with Ipratropium bromide (250mcg) for first 2 h; review frequently. • Consider early single bolus dose of intravenous salbutamol where child has responded poorly to inhaled therapy • Oral steroids: 20 mg prednisolone (2 to 5 years); 30 to 40 mg (> 5 years). Repeat dose if vomiting or consider intravenous steroids (hydrocortisone 4 mg kg^{-1} every 4 h) • Consider aminophylline if child unresponsive to maximal doses of bronchodilators and steroids • Intravenous magnesium is a safe but as yet unproven therapy for acute asthma • Consider ABG if poor response to early treatment

Figure 10.1 Early management of asthma – September 2015. Based on the British Thoracic Society, Scottish Intercollegiate Guidelines Network, British guideline on the management of asthma, revised October 2014

Doses can be repeated at regular intervals. Severe attacks may even necessitate continuous nebulised short-acting beta-2 agonists (e.g. salbutamol). Use oxygen to drive the nebuliser unit (there will be an optimal flow rate to drive the nebuliser to generate the optimal particle size, often 10 to 12 L min^{-1}). Alternatively salbutamol can also be given by a metered dose inhaler and a large volume spacer (for children with moderate asthma this may be equally effective). In near-fatal asthma hypoventilation may prevent effective delivery of nebulised drugs, necessitating the use of intravenous bronchodilation.

o **Steroids:** asthma is an inflammatory disorder and steroids are mandatory for treatment. Give steroids early either intravenous or oral.

o **Nebulised anticholinergics:** (e.g. ipratropium) may produce additional bronchodilation.

o **Magnesium:** a single dose of IV Magnesium sulfate can be given in acute severe asthma not responding to inhaled bronchodilator therapy. Give IV Magnesium as a slow bolus to diminish the risk of hypotension.

o **Aminophylline:** IV aminophylline may give additional benefit for children with severe or life-threatening asthma. It is given as a loading dose, followed by a continuous infusion. Serum concentrations should be monitored (below 20 mcg mL^{-1}) to avoid toxicity.

Illnesses affecting the circulation

Anaphylaxis

Anaphylaxis is a rare but life-threatening generalised or systemic hypersensitivity reaction involving several systems. The most common causes are medications (e.g. antibiotics, aspirin, non-steroidal anti-inflammatory drugs), latex, stinging insects (e.g. wasps, bees) and food (e.g. seafood, peanuts). Anaphylaxis should be considered when two or more systems are affected, predominant ones being involved include cutaneous, respiratory, cardiovascular, neurological or gastrointestinal systems.

- **Airway** – This is at risk of becoming obstructed. The child may have a stridor and signs of respiratory failure due to laryngeal oedema and soft-tissue swelling (i.e. swelling lips and tongue).

- **Breathing** – Respiratory failure may also be due to bronchospasm.

- **Circulation** – Vasodilation causes relative hypovolaemia and increased capillary permeability with extravasation of intravascular fluids into surrounding tissues.

- **Disability** – Decompensated circulatory and/or respiratory failure can lead to a decreasing level of consciousness and is a worrying sign.

- **Exposure** – Flushing, pallor, urticaria.

Management (Figure 10.2)

1. Remove the likely allergen (e.g. antibiotics, blood transfusion).

2. Open the airway.

3. Give 100% O$_2$ with BMV if required. Consider early intubation, particularly in children with lingual, labial and oropharyngeal swelling, and with hoarseness. Early involvement of an experienced anaesthetist is important, as it may be a progressive condition, hence airway management before its total obstruction is an absolute must.

4. Give adrenaline intramuscularly to all children with signs of airway swelling, breathing difficulty or circulatory failure (Figure 10.2). Repeat adrenaline in 5 min if there is no clinical improvement.

5. If the child's clinical manifestations do not respond to medications give 20 mL kg^{-1} IV crystalloid (Chapter 6).

6. Give chlorphenamine (antihistamine):

< 6 months	250 mcg kg^{-1} IM or slow IV
6 months–6 years	2.5 mg IM or slow IV
6–12 years	5 mg IM or slow IV
> 12 years	10 mg IM or slow IV

7. For severe or recurrent reactions and patients with asthma, give hydrocortisone:

< 6 months	25 mg IM or slow IV
6 months–6 years	50 mg IM or slow IV
6–12 years	100 mg IM or slow IV
> 12 years	200 mg IM or slow IV

Children with cardiac problems

Cardiac problems are relatively common (6–8 per 1000 live births) and may present throughout childhood, although most commonly in the neonatal period. Clinical features include the presence of a murmur plus or minus cyanosis. There may also be signs of cardiac failure, such as tachypnoea, crackles on lung auscultation and hepatomegaly and/or poor systemic perfusion such as prolonged CRT, poor or absent pulses and hypotension.

Cardiac problems can be classified as:

1. Congenital cardiac problems including cyanotic (e.g. transposition of great arteries), obstructive (e.g. coarctation of aorta) and hypoplastic (e.g. hypoplastic

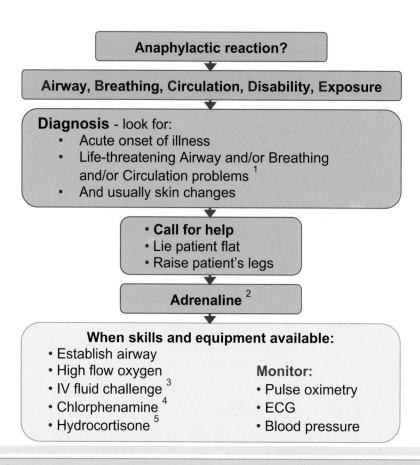

Anaphylactic reaction?

Airway, Breathing, Circulation, Disability, Exposure

Diagnosis - look for:
- Acute onset of illness
- Life-threatening Airway and/or Breathing and/or Circulation problems [1]
- And usually skin changes

- **Call for help**
- Lie patient flat
- Raise patient's legs

Adrenaline [2]

When skills and equipment available:
- Establish airway
- High flow oxygen
- IV fluid challenge [3]
- Chlorphenamine [4]
- Hydrocortisone [5]

Monitor:
- Pulse oximetry
- ECG
- Blood pressure

[1] **Life-threatening problems:**
Airway: swelling, hoarseness, stridor
Breathing: rapid breathing, wheeze, fatigue, cyanosis, SpO_2 < 92%, confusion
Circulation: pale, clammy, low blood pressure, faintness, drowsy/coma

[2] **Adrenaline** *(give IM unless experienced with IV adrenaline)*
IM doses of 1:1000 adrenaline (repeat after 5 min if no better)
- Adult 500 micrograms IM (0.5 mL)
- Child more than 12 years: 500 micrograms IM (0.5 mL)
- Child 6 -12 years: 300 micrograms IM (0.3 mL)
- Child less than 6 years: 150 micrograms IM (0.15 mL)

Adrenaline IV to be given **only by experienced specialists**
Titrate: Adults 50 micrograms; Children 1 microgram/kg

[3] **IV fluid challenge:**
Adult - 500 – 1000 mL
Child - crystalloid 20 mL/kg

Stop IV colloid
if this might be the cause
of anaphylaxis

	[4] Chlorphenamine (IM or slow IV)	[5] Hydrocortisone (IM or slow IV)
Adult or child more than 12 years	10 mg	200 mg
Child 6 - 12 years	5 mg	100 mg
Child 6 months to 6 years	2.5 mg	50 mg
Child less than 6 months	250 micrograms/kg	25 mg

Figure 10.2 Anaphylaxis algorithm

left heart) lesions. When these babies present unexpectedly in the neonatal period, a prostaglandin infusion such as dinoprostone, PGE2, is usually required to open and keep open the ductus arteriosus. Other congenital cardiac lesions include septal defects (e.g. ventricular septal defects, (VSD)) which are generally less severe, present later (usually 6 weeks of age onwards) and do not require prostaglandin. VSDs are the most common form of congenital heart disease (25–30% of cases) and the infants usually present in cardiac failure with signs including tachypnoea, tachycardia, poor perfusion, pallor, hepatomegaly, and crackles in the lung bases and additionally with failure to thrive.

2. Later onset, acquired problems (e.g. myocarditis, cardiomyopathy), usually present with features of cardiac failure with signs including tachycardia, tachypnoea and hepatomegaly.

3. Rhythm disturbance (Chapter 6).

- **Airway** – This is safe if consciousness is not compromised.

- **Breathing** – Several key clinical features include tachypneoa (cardiac failure) and low saturations (particularly cyanotic congenital lesions). A cyanotic congenital cardiac problem is suspected if there is no improvement in saturations when oxygen is administered. In older children with an established cardiac diagnosis, it is helpful to establish and target usual O_2 saturations for them. In heart failure there may be crepitations at the lung bases on auscultation.

- **Circulation** – There may be signs of circulatory compromise or even shock, such as tachycardia, poor peripheral pulses, prolonged capillary refill time and possible hypotension. Other problems such as poor feeding or sepsis may lead to hypovolaemia and fluid boluses may be required but these should be given with caution (see below). An infusion of prostaglandin should be commenced if a neonate is suspected of having a congenital cardiac problem.

- **Disability** – An abnormal conscious level may reflect impaired end-organ function due to respiratory or circulatory compromise. Hypoglycaemia is more likely in a sick infant. Monitor electrolytes particularly if the child is receiving diuretics or drugs to manage cardiac failure.

- **Exposure** – Skin perfusion should be assessed. Although fever may be related to prostaglandin infusion, consider the possibility of sepsis if fever is present.

Management

1. Get senior help immediately.

2. Give high-flow oxygen especially when the diagnosis is uncertain. A brief period of oxygen is unlikely to close a patent ductus arteriosus. Discuss with a paediatric cardiologist as soon as possible.

3. Start a prostaglandin infusion when a neonatal duct dependent problem is suspected (e.g. in cases of sudden unexplained deterioration in the first week or so after birth). Duct-dependent lesions may be due to congenital cyanotic, obstructive or hypoplastic cardiac conditions. Prostaglandin infusions can be given peripherally, or via a dedicated intraosseous line, but should not be given by bolus. Higher doses may cause apnoea requiring respiratory support.

4. Cautious use of diuretics may be helpful in cardiac failure (e.g. VSD) and additional respiratory support may be required.

5. Consider cautious fluid resuscitation using boluses of 10 mL kg^{-1} of 0.9% saline. Carefully reassess after each bolus as worsening tachycardia or liver enlargement suggest fluid overload and then diuretics rather than fluid resuscitation would be indicated.

6. Discuss management with a paediatric cardiologist or intensivist as more sophisticated monitoring (e.g. invasive blood pressure) and therapy (e.g. vasoactive drugs) as well as transfer to a specialist centre, may be required.

Sepsis

Sepsis is a common cause of death in children. It may be accompanied by organ dysfunction (severe sepsis) or hypotension (septic shock). Prompt recognition and management is required (Figure 10.3). Sepsis is diagnosed if there is suspected or proven evidence of infection as the cause of the acute illness *plus at least two of the following*: core temperature < 36 °C or > 38.5 °C; inappropriate tachycardia; altered mental state; reduced peripheral perfusion; white blood cell count <4 or > 12 x 10^9 L^{-1}.

- **Airway** – This may be compromised by reduced level of consciousness (e.g. meningitis, any infection causing shock).

- **Breathing** – Children may have respiratory distress (tachypnoea, increased work of breathing) or respiratory failure due to the underlying condition (pneumonia) or as a result of other processes (septic response). Ventilatory support may be required.

- **Circulation** – Children may have tachycardia, prolonged capillary refill time, poor peripheral pulses and possibly hypotension (cold shock). Sometimes sepsis results in vasodilatation with warm peripheries and early hypotension (warm shock). Fluid maldistribution is common and severe sepsis often additionally causes myocardial dysfunction. Compensated circulatory failure may mask the true severity of the illness and urgency required in management. Careful assessment is required.

- **Disability** – An abnormal conscious level may reflect impaired end-organ function due to respiratory or circulatory compromise. However, abnormal neurological status may reflect the underlying

Recognition Sepsis: Time 0

- **A, B assessment** – airway, RR, work of breathing, oxygen saturations, breath sounds; recognition respiratory distress/failure; open airway and start high flow O₂ 15 L min⁻¹ or BMV as appropriate.
- **C assessment** – HR, CRT, BP, peripheral and central perfusion, rhythm recognition; recognition circulatory failure/shock; establish IV/IO access (take blood cultures, full blood count, blood glucose, urea and electrolytes, lactate*, blood gas and other bloods as indicated**) and give fluid resuscitation as below.
- **D assessment** – AVPU score; recognition of altered mental status secondary to poor perfusion.
- **E assessment** – rash, temperature (high or low).
- Sepsis is diagnosed if there is evidence of infection as cause of the acute illness (suspected or proven) plus at least two of the following: core temperature < 36 °C or > 38.5 °C; white cell count elevated or depressed for age; inappropriate tachycardia; altered mental state; reduced peripheral perfusion.

Initial resuscitation: Time 5 min

- If no hepatomegaly or rales/crackles then push 20 mL kg⁻¹ 0.9% NaCl iv bolus over 5–10 min and re-assess after each bolus up to 60 ml kg⁻¹ until perfusion improved.
- Therapeutic end points: CRT< 2 s; normal BP for age; UO > 1mL kg⁻¹ hour⁻¹; normal pulses; normal mental state.
- Watch for signs of fluid overload (crackles at lung bases, jugular venousdistension and hepatomegaly); if present **stop** bolus therapy and start inotropic support.
- Correct hypoglycaemia and hypocalcaemia.
- Start broad spectrum antibiotics and seek and aggressively control any infection source.
- Call for more senior help and an anaesthetist urgently; call PICU for bed +/-PICU transfer team.
- If mechanical ventilation is required then cardiovascular instability during intubation is less likely after appropriate cardiovascular resuscitation.

Fluid refractory shock?

Fluid refractory shock: Time 15 - 60 min

- Start peripheral IV/IO inotrope infusion, preferably Adrenaline 0.05-0.3 mcg kg⁻¹ min⁻¹.
- Use ketamine +/-atropine IV/IO/IM to gain central access and airway if needed.
- **Titrate Adrenaline** 0.05 -0.3 mcg kg⁻¹ min⁻¹ for **Cold Shock***.
- (Titrate central Dopamine 5 -9 mcg kg⁻¹ min⁻¹ if adrenaline not available).
- **Titrate central Noradrenaline** from 0.05 mcg kg⁻¹ min⁻¹ and upward to reverse **Warm Shock***.
- (Titrate central Dopamine > 10 mcg kg⁻¹ min⁻¹ if Noradrenaline not available).

Catecholamine-resistant shock?

PICU Team

- Further management as per Paediatric Intensive Care/ retrieval service advice.

Figure 10.3 Early management of severe sepsis in infants and children. Clinical Practice Parameters for Hemodynamic Support of Pediatric and Neonatal Septic Shock. Crit Care Med. 2017;45(6):1061–1093.

condition itself (e.g. meningitis). Blood glucose should always be checked as hypoglycaemia is relatively common and should be rechecked if new problems (e.g. seizures) are encountered.

- **Exposure** – This can give clues to the diagnosis. Look for rashes (e.g. meningococcal disease, toxic shock) or other skin lesions (e.g. herpes simplex).

Management

1. Get senior help immediately.
2. Give 100% oxygen initially. Consider early intubation by an experienced anaesthetist especially if > 40 mL kg⁻¹ of IV fluid has been required.

Intubation is safer if performed when cardiovascular stability has been achieved.

3. Antibiotics should be administered within 1 h of presentation. The choice depends on the suspected site of infection and organism (and resistance pattern if known) – refer to local antibiotic guidelines. Third generation cephalosporins (e.g. cefotaxime) are often appropriate. Consider the possibility of other organisms (e.g. herpes simplex).
4. Fluid resuscitation using boluses of 20 mL kg⁻¹ of 0.9% saline initially. Do not hesitate to use the intraosseous (IO) route. Large quantities of fluid may be required.

Carefully reassess after each bolus. Children with no signs of circulatory failure do not need volume resuscitation. A tachycardia or fever alone is not enough to diagnose circulatory failure.

5. Vasoactive drugs may be required. These IV infusions optimise cardiac output by improving cardiac contractility (inotropes) for example, adrenaline which is the first line inotrope in sepsis; raising systemic vascular resistance for example noradrenaline or raising the heart rate (chronotropes). They should be considered in children especially where shock is unresponsive to fluid boluses (i.e. after 40–60 mL kg^{-1} fluid bolus resuscitation). Adrenaline is generally the first line inotrope in children and can be given peripherally; other vasoactive drugs can initially be administered by the IO route until central access is secured (Chapter 5).

6. Seek specialist advice early as more sophisticated monitoring (e.g. invasive blood pressure), management decisions (blood product use) and adjunctive treatments may be required.

Illnesses affecting the central nervous system

Coma – The child with a diminished level of consciousness

A child's conscious level may be altered by illness, injury or intoxication. The level of awareness decreases from alert (A) to stages of drowsiness (mild reduction in alertness and increase in hours of sleep) but responsive to voice (V), to responsive only to pain (P), and finally to unconsciousness (U) (unrousable/unresponsive).

- **Airway** – As the child's level of consciousness diminishes, the likelihood of obstruction of the airway increases owing to the loss of tone of soft tissue and supporting musculature. When the child becomes reactive only to pain, there may be loss of protective cough and gag reflex, hence aspiration of stomach contents may occur.

- **Breathing** – Coma may lead to slow respiratory rate and/or inadequate respiratory effort.

- **Circulation** – Depending upon the cause of the coma, circulation can be affected (e.g. hypovolaemic shock in septic shock, hypovolaemic shock in trauma) and should be managed accordingly.

- **Disability** – The assessment is based on AVPU, posture and pupil reaction. Recording these values is essential and form part of the ongoing assessment and management of the child. After the initial assessment of ABCDE with interventions being carried out, more detailed neurological assessment is required to determine the cause of the change in the level of consciousness.

- **Exposure** – Causes such as meningococcaemia or other infective causes (e.g. vasculitis, SLE) may cause a decreased conscious level. The associated dermal manifestations can help make the diagnosis.

Management

Open the airway and maintain its patency by appropriate means (e.g. airway opening manoeuvres, nasopharyngeal or oropharyngeal airway adjuncts, or tracheal intubation may be required).

If protection against aspiration is required because of loss of the protective upper airway reflexes, intubation must be performed by rapid sequence induction of anaesthesia. Ventilatory support will then be required.

Call for help early if a decreased level of consciousness is diagnosed. The following points have been adapted from the RCPCH 2015 guidelines for the management of a child with decreased conscious level:

- Always consider raised intracranial pressure and look for the signs: A and B – abnormal breathing, C – bradycardia and hypertension (MAP > 95th centile), D – pupil(s) dilated and loss of light reaction, posturing.

- Neuroimaging will likely be indicated either CT or MRI brain.

- If toxins are suspected then urine and blood samples should be collected early and sent for toxicology.

- If fits are prolonged despite anticonvulsant therapy consider further investigations (e.g. electroencephalogram (EEG)), metabolic tests including blood glucose).

- Involve PICU and/or neurosurgeons for advice early.

- Treatments are beyond the scope of this algorithm, refer to local protocols RCPCH and NICE guidelines.

Seizures

Seizures are the most common paediatric emergency. The neurological status should be assessed and treated after airway, breathing, and circulation have been assessed and managed, as these are the initial priority. However in many cases A, B and C may improve only once the seizures have been treated.

There are many causes of seizures in children and infants (e.g. idiopathic epilepsy, structural brain abnormalities, traumatic brain injury, bleeds and thrombosis in the brain, febrile convulsions, metabolic disorders, intoxications, meningitis and encephalitis). There are some biochemical disturbances that can also cause seizures including: hypoglycaemia (common in children and infants), severe hyponatraemia, hypocalcaemia and hypomagnesaemia.

A generalised seizure that has been ongoing for five minutes is unlikely to terminate without active management. When seizures have continued for 30 min or more this is known as convulsive status epilepticus.

Time 0 min
- Seizure starts; confirm clinically
- Check ABC, high flow O_2
- Check blood glucose, treat < 3 mmol L^{-1}

Time 5 min
- **Midazolam** 0.3–0.5 mg kg^{-1} bucally*

  OR
- **Lorazepam** 0.1 mg kg^{-1} IV or IO

Time 15 min
- **Lorazepam** 0.1 mg kg^{-1} IV
- (Reconfirm epileptic seizure and prepare phenytoin for next step)

Time 25 min
- **Phenytoin** 20 mg kg^{-1} by intravenous infusion over 20 min,

  OR (if on regular phenytoin already)
- **Phenobarbital** 20 mg kg^{-1} by intravenous infusion over 5 min

Time 45 min
- Rapid sequence induction of anaesthesia using **thiopental sodium** 4 mg kg^{-1} intravenously
- Intubation

*See BNFc for exact age related doses

Figure 10.4 Management of status epilepticus – September 2015. Adapted from NICE guidelines for treating convulsive status epilepticus in children (2011)

- **Airway** – This is at risk of becoming or can be obstructed during a fit. This may be due to secretions or tongue/soft tissue hypotonia, with loss of the protective upper airway reflexes.

- **Breathing** – Respiratory failure is due to airway obstruction or a decreased level of consciousness slowing the respiratory rate. Respiratory arrest can occur due to central nervous system depression; this is more likely if the child is receiving antiepileptic drugs (e.g. benzodiazepines) in the emergency treatment of seizures because they have respiratory depressant side effects.

- **Circulation** – This is generally normal until decompensated respiratory failure. However, if the aetiology of the seizure is associated with other diseases (e.g. meningococcal disease or head trauma), circulatory failure may present earlier.

- **Disability** – Seizures should be controlled by antiepileptic drugs according to national guidelines. The first-line therapy is a benzodiazepine (diazepam, midazolam or lorazepam) – but only two doses (if required) should be administered. The blood glucose level should always be measured as hypoglycaemia is a treatable cause. Blood glucose levels < 3 mmol L^{-1} should be treated with 2 mL kg^{-1} 10% dextrose bolus. Other blood tests should be as directed by aetiology of condition.

- **Exposure** – As with coma, the skin may reveal the cause for the seizure such as infective causes, neurocutaneous disorders or other disorders, and help specialists in determining further management.

Management

Open the airway and maintain patency by appropriate means. Treat seizures according to national (Figure 10.4. A guideline for early management of status epilepticus based on NICE guidelines), local or the child's own guidelines (children and infants with known seizures may have their own protocols developed by their neurologist).

If the child remains hypoxic after airway opening, BMV with oxygen should be performed. Tracheal intubation and ventilation may sometimes be necessary to protect the airway and prevent aspiration of stomach contents. Respiratory depression after benzodiazepine administration is common and the child or infant may require respiratory support for a period of time after cessation of status epilepticus, this should be anticipated and senior help sought.

In septic patients consider measuring calcium and magnesium levels as they are sometimes low.

Illnesses affecting metabolic and electrolyte balance

Some electrolyte disturbances can cause cardiac arrhythmias, cardiorespiratory arrest or can make resuscitation less effective.

In some circumstances the correction of an anticipated electrolyte disturbance may be started, based on clinical parameters, before laboratory results are available.

Diabetic ketoacidosis

Diabetic ketoacidosis (DKA) is caused by low insulin levels and associated increase in other hormones such as glucagon, cortisol and growth hormone. This results in the following key features of DKA:

- hyperglycaemia (blood glucose > 11 mmol L^{-1})
- hypersomolality
- ketonaemia
- metabolic acidosis (pH < 7.3, bicarbonate < 18 mmol L^{-1})

Clinical features include dehydration, abnormal deep sighing respiration (Kussmaul breaths), vomiting and drowsiness. The clinical history may include increased urine output, increased thirst, weight loss, abdominal pain and confusion.

Do not overestimate the degree of dehydration. A guide is outlined in Table 10.1.

Table 10.1 Dehydration guide

Degree Dehydration	
5–10% mild to moderate	pH 7.1 and above
> 10% severe	pH < 7.1

DKA can be fatal. Cerebral oedema accounts for 57–87% of all DKA deaths. Other causes include aspiration pneumonia and hypokalaemia. Because of this it is important to recognise DKA early and get senior help. The aim is to rehydrate but minimise the risk of cerebral oedema.

- **Airway** – This is safe if consciousness is not compromised but careful assessment is required in the presence of altered level of consciousness.

- **Breathing** – Children are often breathing quickly to compensate for their metabolic acidosis. Avoid intubation if at all possible.

- **Circulation** – Assess for signs of circulatory failure. Signs of shock are very rare but can occur and include poor peripheral pulses, CRT and hypotension.

- **Disability** – Assess level of consciousness using GCS score or AVPU. Continue hourly neurological observations looking for signs of raised intracranial pressure (e.g. posturing, falling GCS score, rising BP with bradycardia, unequal or poorly reactive pupils). Monitor blood glucose, sodium and potassium.

- **Exposure** – Fever is not a feature of DKA. If present, take blood cultures and consider antibiotics.

Management

1. Admit to high dependency bed if pH < 7.1 and/or child < 2 years.

2. Admit to paediatric intensive care if blood glucose > 50 mmol L^{-1} and or persistent shock and/or signs raised ICP.

3. Ensure the airway is patent.

4. Intubation should be avoided unless the patient has a GCS < 8, has a respiratory arrest or has poor respiratory effort. Intubation and ventilation is dangerous as the children often have a low pH due to the metabolic acidosis, which they are compensating for by hyperventilating with a low pCO_2. After intubation the pCO_2 almost always rises causing a further drop in pH which might precipitate cardiorespiratory arrest.

5. Insert a nasogastric tube to prevent aspiration of vomit.

6. Obtain vascular access and check blood gases (pH, pCO_2, bicarbonate), blood sugar, urea and electrolytes including serum potassium and serum beta-hydroxybutyrate. Attach a cardiac monitor. If CRT > 2 s and other signs of shock give 10 mL kg^{-1} 0.9% saline and reassess. Repeat to a maximum of 20 mL kg^{-1}, ask for senior assistance and inform PICU if shock persists.

7. Do not give bicarbonate as its use is associated with an increased risk of cerebral oedema.

8. Assess the degree of dehydration. The aim is to correct the dehydration slowly over 48 h with maintenance fluids plus deficit calculated from degree of dehydration. If pH < 7.1 commence IV fluids with 0.9% saline; add potassium once renal failure excluded. Management based on British Society for Paediatric Endocrinology and Diabetes (BSPED) guidelines is given in Figure 10.5.

9. If there are any signs of reduced conscious level or raised intracranial pressure assume that the patient has cerebral oedema. Get senior help immediately.

10. Start insulin infusion approximately one hour after maintenance fluids and replacement fluids started, as per protocol, at 0.05–0.1 U kg^{-1} h^{-1}.

Identify DKA	• Blood glucose > 11 mmol L^{-1} • pH < 7.3 • Bicarbonate < 18 mmol L^{-1} • Ketones: blood beta-hydroxybutyrate > 3mmol L^{-1} or urine ketonuria ++ and above • History polyuria, polydipsia, weight loss, vomiting, excessive tiredness, confusion, abdominal pain, hyperventilation • Note: Usually not vomiting, acidotic or drowsy unless more than 5% dehydrated • Assess dehydration and conscious level

> **HDU: pH < 7.1 and/or child < 2 years**
> **PICU: blood glucose > 50 mmol L^{-1} and or persistent shock and/or signs raised ICP**

Resuscitation	**A** ensure airway patency, insert NG tube if reduced conscious level or vomiting **B** 100% oxygen via facemask with reservoir bag + titrate to oxygen saturations 94-98%; avoid intubation unless respiratory arrest or respiratory failure when senior help urgently required **C** establish IV access, take bloods (pH, pCO$_2$, bicarbonate, sodium, potassium, urea, beta-hydroxybutyrate levels, glucose) monitor ECG, identify shock – this is **very** unusual in DKA • If pH < 7.1 plus signs shock CRT > 2 s, low BP +/- reduced LOC give 10 mL kg^{-1} and reassess; repeat to a maximum of 20 mL kg^{-1} – ask for senior assistance and inform PICU if shock is persists **D** identify signs raised intracranial pressure – posturing, falling GCS, rising BP with bradycardia and if present inform PICU **E** Consider sepsis if fever, hypothermia, hypotension, lactic acisosis, refractory acidosis

Intravenous therapy: fluids and insulin	• For: children with nausea and vomiting, or reduced conscious level or clinically severe dehydration • Aim: to correct marked dehydration slowly over 48 h; calculate fluid requirements (FR) • FR = Maintenance fluids for 48 h + (estimated fluid deficit) • 0.9% saline initial fluid of choice - add potassium once passing urine • 1–2 h after intravenous fluids commenced start insulin infusion at 0.05–0.1 units kg^{-1} h^{-1} • **Do not give intravenous bicarbonate to correct acidosis**

Observations	• Hourly blood glucose (avoid reduction in > 5 mmol L^{-1} hr^{-1}) • Neurological observations (every 30 to 60 min), fluid balance, weight, BP, HR, RR, temperature • Initially two hourly U+E's, blood gas, blood ketones +/- urine ketones • Serum sodium level should rise, not fall and therapy can be guided by corrected serum sodium levels • When blood glucose < 14 mmol L^{-1} use 0.9% saline with 5% dextrose with added potassium (KCl 40 mmol L^{-1}) as fluid therapy

Maintenance Fluids in DKA: lower than standard because large volumes associated with increased risk of cerebral oedema	
Weight	**Maintenance Fluid rate**
< 10 kg	2 mL kg^{-1} hour^{-1}
10–40 kg	1 mL kg^{-1} hour^{-1}
> 40 kg	40 mL hour^{-1}
Fluid deficit (mL) = % dehydration x weight (kg) x 10	
Fluid requirement (FR) over 48 h = Maintenance requirement for 48 h + (fluid deficit – resuscitation fluid given*) * Volume of fluid used for resuscitation only deducted if > 20 mL kg^{-1}	**e.g. 10 kg child,** 10% dehydrated resuscitated with 10 mL kg^{-1} 0.9% saline = (1 x 10 x 48) + (10 x 10 x 10) = 1480 mL over 48 h = 31 mL h^{-1}
Corrected Na = Na + 0.4 (glucose) – 5.5 mmol L^{-1}	

Mortality in childhood DKA
Cerebral oedema
	Unpredictable. Higher risk in severe acidosis, young child and first presentation. Mortality ≈ 25%. Avoid by slow correction of metabolic disturbance.
	Assume cerebral oedema if:
	  • reduced level of conscious
	  • abnormalities in breathing pattern (e.g. respiratory pauses)
	  • oculomotor palsies
	  • pupillary inequality or dilatation
	Treat with: 20% mannitol 0.5–1 g kg^{-1} over 10 to 15 mins IV
	Or
	2.7% or 3% hypertonic saline 2.5–5 ml kg^{-1} over 10 to 15 min IV

Hypokalaemia	This is preventable with careful monitoring and management.
Aspiration pneumonia	Use a naso-gastric tube in semi-conscious or unconscious children.

Figure 10.5 Adapted NICE guidelines August 2015 (updated November 2016) NG18.

Sodium (Na⁺)

Sodium is the major cation (positive ion) in the extracellular, and hence intravascular, fluid compartment. Hence the sodium concentration in the blood largely determines plasma tonicity (osmolality). Disturbances in sodium levels can cause or occur due to fluid shifts between the different fluid compartments in the body disrupting homeostasis and disturbing cellular function.

Hyponatraemia

The normal range of sodium in the blood is 135–145 mmol L^{-1} and hyponatraemia is defined as serum sodium < 135 mmol L^{-1}. Hyponatraemia can develop because of excess free water intake, excessive loss of sodium from the kidney or gastrointestinal tract, retention of free water by the kidney, but rarely deficient intake of sodium.

Plasma tonicity is fiercely defended by the body because of its importance in maintaining homeostasis and usually the body can maintain serum sodium in the normal range despite wide variations in fluid ingestion. This is achieved by the kidney's ability to generate dilute urine and excrete free water in response to changes in serum osmolality and intravascular volume status. A hormone called anti-diuretic hormone (ADH) is secreted from the pituitary when the body detects a high blood tonicity or low blood volume. This hormone acts on the kidney making it conserve water in order to increase intravascular volume.

In most children hyponatraemia is acquired during hospitalisation. The reasons for this are two-fold. Firstly, particularly sick children are unable to handle water normally as they can develop the syndrome of inappropriate anti-diuretic hormone (SIADH). In this scenario the ADH hormone is secreted even though plasma tonicity and or blood volume are normal or high and this can result in hyponatraemia. This may be further exacerbated if hypotonic fluids are used as intravenous fluid therapy. Triggers for SIADH include morphine, ventilation, intracranial conditions, pneumonia, asthma and barbiturates. This is why sick children in PICU are often fluid restricted and not given full maintenance fluids.

Other conditions that can lead to hyponatraemia include heart failure and nephrotic syndrome (where there is increased total body water); diuretic use and reduced sodium intake; loss of sodium via the gastrointestinal or urinary tract (cerebral salt wasting, gastroenteritis, fistulas).

Most of the signs and symptoms of hyponatraemia occur because of its effects on the central nervous system. When serum sodium and hence blood osmolality falls, water enters the brain causing cerebral oedema. Cerebral oedema is the cause of symptoms such as headache, nausea, vomiting, irritability and seizures. Symptoms can vary depending upon how quickly the hyponatraemia developed, the level of sodium reached and the duration of the hyponatraemia. Seizures are very unusual at sodium levels > 125 mmol L^{-1} and become increasingly common at levels below 120 mmol L^{-1}. Other signs and symptoms include tachycardia, muscle cramps, hypotension and muscle weakness.

Management

- **Airway** – not usually compromised unless reduced level of consciousness or seizures.

- **Breathing** – may have reduced respiratory rate if reduced level of consciousness.

- **Circulation** – obtain vascular access and measure blood electrolytes. In hypovolaemic hyponatraemia states may need to give fluid resuscitation to restore haemodynamic stability, thereafter sodium should be corrected slowly at a rate of increase of not more than 0.5 mmol L^{-1} h^{-1}.

- **Disability** – if sodium level is < 125 mmol L^{-1} and the patient is seizing then the sodium level should be corrected to 125 mmol L^{-1} as this would treat any seizures related to hyponatraemia. If the seizures are continuing then other causes should be sought. Treatment is with 3mL kg^{-1} of 3% saline given over 20 min.

For hyponatraemia associated with euvolaemia or hypervolaemia fluid restriction and or diuretics may be useful. Again the serum sodium should be corrected slowly at a rate of change no more than 0.5 mmol L^{-1} h^{-1}. This becomes increasingly important the more chronic the hyponatraemia is because when it develops slowly there is a slow cerebral adaptation to protect the brain from the injurious effects of hypo-osmolality. This protective mechanism leaves the brain susceptible to demyelination syndrome during treatment if the correction is rapid. Further management is directed at finding and correcting the underlying cause.

Hypernatraemia

Hypernatraemia is defined as serum sodium > 145 mmol L^{-1}. It represents a deficit of total body water relative to total body sodium levels. It is commonly caused by loss of free water but can also be caused by excessive salt administration.

Plasma tonicity is increased in hypernatraemia and this causes cellular dehydration.

The brain is particularly vulnerable to these effects and cell shrinkage can result in seizures and encephalopathy and tearing of cerebral blood vessels causing haemorrhage.

Most at risk are critically ill children, those who are neurologically impaired and infants who are unable to respond to their thirst trigger.

Causes include:

- water depletion (e.g. diabetes insipidus)

- water depletion exceeding sodium depletion (e.g. gastroenteritis and diarrhoea, breast feeding failure)

- sodium excess (e.g. administration of hypertonic solutions, infant formula made up incorrectly).

Signs and symptoms are more common at serum sodium levels of > 160 mmol L^{-1} and are more common when hypernatraemia develops acutely.

They include: irritability, lethargy, altered level of consciousness, seizures, ataxia, tremor, hyperreflexia, increased muscle tone and fever. Severe hypernatraemia occurs at serum sodium levels of > 170 mmol L^{-1}.

Management

- **Airway** – not usually compromised unless reduced level of consciousness or seizures.

- **Breathing** – may have reduced respiratory rate if reduced level of consciousness.

- **Circulation** – obtain vascular access and measure blood electrolytes. In hypovolaemic hypernatraemia states may need to give fluid resuscitation to restore haemodynamic stability, thereafter sodium should be corrected slowly at a rate of decrease of not more than 0.5 mmol L^{-1} h^{-1}.

Rehydration should be over 48 to 72 h because rapid rehydration of prolonged hypernatraemia states (with rapid decreases in serum sodium levels) will result in cerebral oedema. In severe hypernatraemia, levels in excess 170 mmol L^{-1}, 0.9% saline should be used to rehydrate and potassium added once the patient is passing urine. Further management should be directed at finding and correcting any cause.

Potassium (K$^+$)

The causes of hyperkalaemia and hypokalaemia are given in Table 10.2.

The K$^+$ gradient, from the intracellular to extracellular space, determines the conduction of the myocardial cells and therefore their contractility. Even limited increases in serum K$^+$ can be responsible for decreased conduction and diminished cardiac contractility. Arterial pH has a direct effect on K$^+$; acidosis increases serum K$^+$ (by 0.5–1.1 mmol L^{-1} for each 0.1 decrease in pH).

Table 10.2 Causes of potassium disturbance	
Hyperkalaemia	**Hypokalaemia**
Renal failure (acute/chronic)	Gastrointestinal losses (e.g. diarrhoea, vomiting)
Acidosis Adrenal insufficiency • Addison's disease • Secondary	Alkalosis
Excessive potassium intake	Volume depletion
Intake of K$^+$ sparing medication	Diuretics
Cell lysis (e.g. in tumour treatment, tissue infarction)	Insufficient potassium intake
Haemolysis	Malnutrition
Massive blood transfusions	Insufficient K$^+$ intake

Hyperkalaemia

Hyperkalaemia (K$^+$ > 7 mmol L^{-1}) is characterised by muscular weakness, paralytic ileus, respiratory arrest and heart conduction disturbances leading to arrhythmias and eventually to cardiac arrest.

Typical ECG changes seen in hyperkalaemia are dependent on both the K$^+$ level and the associated rate of increase in K$^+$ level.

Initially there is T wave elevation but this progresses into an idioventricular rhythm and ventricular fibrillation as serum K$^+$ rises.

False hyperkalaemia values can result from haemolysis of the blood due to difficult capillary blood sampling.

Management

The treatment of hyperkalaemia is dependent on the speed of occurrence of the symptoms and the clinical state of the child, or if they show toxic ECG changes. It includes:

1. Intravenous calcium chloride or calcium gluconate is given as a bolus, or over 2–5 min if the child is not in cardiorespiratory arrest to antagonise the toxic effects of hyperkalaemia at the myocardial cell membrane.

2. Sodium bicarbonate (if acidosis or renal failure is present).

3. Insulin-glucose infusion.

4. Salbutamol administration either via a nebuliser or intravenously.

5. Haemodialysis/peritoneal dialysis.

If the child shows elevation of the serum K$^+$ levels only with no symptoms, excess K$^+$ may be removed from the body by the use of:

1. Diuretics (e.g. furosemide).

2. Ion exchange resins (calcium resonium given orally or rectally). Onset of the effect is slow but this treatment can be started early (as soon as the K$^+$ level is increased).

Hypokalaemia

Hypokalaemia (K$^+$ < 3.5 mmol L^{-1}) is characterised by muscular weakness, constipation, paresthesia and tetany.

Severe hypokalaemia (< 2.5 mmol L^{-1}) can cause life-threatening arrhythmias (VF, pVT, PEA or asystole), paralysis, rhabdomyolysis, paralytic ileus and metabolic alkalosis.

Management

Treatment of hypokalaemia (2.5–3.5 mmol L^{-1}) includes the early recognition of the cause. Patients treated with digitalis are at special risk of developing arrhythmias.

Treatment of severe hypokalaemia (< 2.5 mmol L^{-1}) or hypokalaemia associated with arrhythmias consists of careful intravenous K$^+$ infusion (preferably via central access) under ECG monitoring.

This is best performed in a high dependency or PICU setting as arrhythmias can occur. An infusion of 0.5 mmol kg^{-1} h^{-1} of KCl is given until the arrhythmia resolves and/or the K$^+$ level is > 3.5 mmol L^{-1}. A total dose of 2–3 mmol kg^{-1} KCl may be required; administration of K$^+$ should be reduced as soon as the child is clinically stable.

Calcium

Hypercalcaemia

Hypercalcaemia usually presents as long-standing anorexia, malaise, weight loss, failure to thrive and vomiting. Other symptoms are convulsions, coma, polyuria, dehydration, hypokalaemia, bradycardia, arterial hypertension and ECG changes (e.g. short QT, widening of QRS complexes, AV block).

Causes include:

- hyperparathyroidism

- hypervitaminosis A or D

- idiopathic hypercalcaemia of infancy

- malignancy

- thiazide diuretic abuse

- skeletal disorders.

Management

Treatment of hypercalcaemia is mandatory when symptoms appear.

Initial treatment consists of fluid resuscitation with 0.9% saline. Infusion of twice the calculated basic requirement is delivered, providing the degree of dehydration, cardiac function and blood pressure permit significant fluid administration. Levels of both serum K$^+$ and magnesium (Mg^{2+}) should be monitored. Furosemide can be useful in patients with fluid overload; however, in children with renal insufficiency and oliguria, dialysis is necessary.

Hypocalcaemia

Causes include:

- hypoparathyroidism (di George syndrome, magnesium deficiency, familial)

- vitamin D deficiency

- vitamin D resistance

- hypoproteinaemia

- phosphate intoxication.

Specific symptoms are:

- signs of neuronal irritation

- convulsions

- laryngeal stridor

- rickets

- ECG changes: QT prolongation, AV block, VF.

Non-specific symptoms are vomiting, muscular weakness and irritability.

Management

The treatment of severe hypocalcaemia (without hypomagnesaemia) includes intravenous or intraosseous administration of calcium gluconate. Oral supplements of calcium may be needed.

If hypocalcaemia is associated with hypomagnaesemia, Mg^{2+} replacement will also be necessary.

Summary learning

- **The conditions described in this chapter are common causes of paediatric illness and potential causes of cardiorespiratory arrest in children.**
- **Use the ABCDE approach for early recognition and treatment to prevent cardiorespiratory arrest.**
- **Call for expert help early when specialist procedures are needed.**

My key take-home messages from this chapter

http://publications.nice.org.uk/guidance/ CG137 Appendix F: Protocols for treating convulsive status epilepticus in children 2011 (updated Dec 2013).

Further reading

ILCOR Worksheets on therapeutic hypothermia.

http://www.americanheart.org

Alberta Medical Association; Alberta Clinical Practice Guideline Working Group. Guideline for the diagnosis and management of croup, 2008.

Resuscitation Council UK guidance on the management of anaphylaxis http://www.resus.org.uk/pages/faqAna.htm

NICE guidelines NG 18 August 2015 (updated November 2016).

Bronchiolitis in Children. NICE Guideline (NG9). June 2015.

British Thoracic Society, Scottish Intercollegiate Guidelines Network British guideline on the management of asthma in Children. October 2014.

Clinical practice Parameters for Hemodynamic Support of Pediatric and Neonatal Septic Shock. Crit Care Med 2017;45(6):1061-1093.

Hoffman JIE, Kaplan S. The incidence of congenital heart disease. Journal of the American College of Cardiology. 2002; 12 (39). 1890-1900.

The injured child

Contents

- Injury patterns in children
- Team assessment of injured child using AcBCDE approach
- Primary and secondary surveys including cervical spine management and haemorrhage management
- Traumatic brain injury management
- Chest, abdominal and skeletal trauma
- Burns, drowning and non-accidental injury

Learning outcomes

To enable you to:

- Describe the AcBCDE approach in trauma
- Understand that the need for a team approach is essential
- Discuss the need for in-line cervical spine immobilisation
- Discuss the importance of primary and secondary surveys
- Identify the priorities in managing head, cervical spine, thoracic, abdominal and limb injuries
- Manage children with burns
- Manage children following drowning

Blunt trauma is seen in 80% of paediatric cases in the UK; of these, two thirds of life-threatening paediatric trauma is related to brain injury. Mortality from trauma is significantly increased if the triad of acidosis, hypothermia and coagulopathy are present.

Injury patterns in children vary from those seen in adults, owing to the different physiological and anatomical responses to trauma. In children, there is a relatively smaller muscle mass, less subcutaneous tissue and increased elasticity of ribs and other bones. This means that in the child more of the impacting energy is transmitted to underlying organs such as the lungs (often without rib fractures) or abdomen (with damage to visceral organs). Internal injury must therefore always be considered as there may have been significant force involved without external signs being present. The history of the mechanism of injury must always be sought and the clinical consequences of how the impacting energy has been dispersed through the child's body must be considered.

The AcBCDE approach in trauma

When dealing with an injured child appropriate resuscitative measures must be carried out as soon as problems are identified. These measures must be applied by an effective team using a structured approach to ensure maximal benefit.

This structured approach involves every team member co-ordinating their activity so the primary survey (AcBCDE) and resuscitation are being performed simultaneously. This is followed by:

- X-ray series: chest and pelvis. Note that the cervical spine X-ray may be deferred as part of the secondary survey. Some centres may choose to perform a trauma CT scan instead, but this is not universal.

- secondary survey

- emergency treatment

- definitive care.

The general principles of resuscitation for the injured child are similar to those of the critically ill child but there are a few important differences which are described in this chapter.

The team approach in trauma

Treatment of trauma in children demands a skilled team that is able to work in parallel while performing dedicated tasks. The team leader, who coordinates the management of the child, should allocate tasks. Ideally team members should have their roles easily identified (e.g. labels on their tops).

The optimal trauma team comprises:

- paediatric emergency medicine specialist

- paediatric trauma nurses

- paediatric anaesthetists

- paediatric intensivist

- paediatric surgeon

- other specialists may be involved particularly after the secondary survey (e.g. neurosurgical opinion).

Whilst this is an optimal major trauma team, it is not always possible. However, senior experienced help must be sought urgently, ideally before the child arrives.

Primary survey

Airway compromise, respiratory failure, circulatory failure and brain injury can co-exist following trauma. The primary survey is a systematic rapid evaluation, which identifies life-threatening problems using the AcBCDE approach. It is completed in the first minutes of the initial assessment of the child.

Resuscitation occurs throughout the primary survey, with problems being treated as soon as they are found: 'treat first what kills first'.

Adhere to the structured process of AcBCDE. 'Distracting' injuries must not interrupt the primary and secondary surveys or life-threatening injuries may be missed. However if there has been life-threatening haemorrhage

Treat first what kills first

Ac **Airway and cervical spine** stabilisation

B **Breathing** oxygenation and ventilation (consider tension pneumothorax)

C **Circulation** and external haemorrhage control

D **Disability** neurological status (AVPU, pupils, posture)

E **Exposure (and Environment)** undress the child, keep them warm and understand the history and consequences of the traumatic event

from the outset then this would be attended to simultaneously with A and B assessment by a trauma team. Monitoring should be attached as soon as possible (SpO$_2$, ECG, BP) during the primary survey.

Ac – Airway and in-line cervical spine immobilisation

Airway

If cervical spine (C-spine) injury is suspected, try to open the airway using the jaw thrust manoeuvre while manually immobilising the cervical spine (Figure 11.1). Opening the airway takes priority, however, and head extension may be necessary; very gently increase the amount of extension until the airway is just open. Clear the oropharynx of debris, blood, vomit and other secretions by gentle suction under direct vision. The neck is inspected for distended veins, tracheal deviation, wounds, or subcutaneous emphysema. It may be necessary to assist the airway by using an oropharyngeal airway, remembering that this will not protect the airway in the event of vomiting, as vomit can be inhaled. If the child tolerates an oropharyngeal airway, this indicates loss of the gag reflex and intubation should be considered. In severe trauma, a tracheal tube is used to secure the airway or, when intubation is not possible, a surgical airway is established.

In-line cervical spine immobilisation

Immobilisation is indicated in high-energy trauma, signs of potential spinal injury and decreased consciousness. If a child is resisting immobilisation and uncooperative they should either be sedated or not immobilised. This is because a distressed and immobilised child is more likely to sustain cervical damage rather than be protected from it.

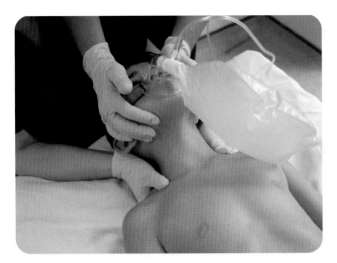

Figure 11.1 Jaw thrust on a child with manual in-line cervical spine immobilisation

If a child is walking they should position themselves on a bed or trolley. Non-ambulant individuals should be placed on a scoop stretcher and should not be placed on extrication boards for more than 30 min. As part of pre-hospital management the child may then be transferred to a vacuum-mattress from the scoop before transfer to hospital depending on urgency. A quick examination of the child's back using a minimum of lateral elevation can be made when the child is placed on the scoop stretcher, therefore avoiding a log-roll.

Regardless of being on a scoop stretcher or in a vacuum-mattress, specific further attention must be paid to in-line C-spine immobilisation. A child, compared to an adult, has a relatively large head, immature vertebral bodies (with less tensile strength) through which the spinal cord travels, strong elastic intervertebral ligaments, flexile joints capsules and easily compressible soft tissue in the neck. As these structures are pliable, injury to the cervical spinal cord, although uncommon, may occur even without radiographic abnormality being seen on either X-ray or CT scan. This is known as spinal cord injury without radiological abnormalities (SCIWORA).

In-line immobilisation of the C-spine can be maintained manually by a single rescuer throughout the on-going resuscitation, although this prevents one rescuer from doing other tasks. As an alternative, to immobilise the C-spine, the use of head blocks (or equivalent) is advocated. These head blocks can be either positioned within the vacuum-mattress or strapped to the scoop stretcher.

There is much controversy concerning the use of cervical collars, especially in children. Cervical collars might induce problems in airway management or cerebral perfusion. There is no proof of their added value in terms of preventing further C-spine injury, especially if the collar does not fit well as is often the case in children. Therefore the standard use of collars is no longer advised. Collars might still have a place during the extraction of a severely injured child or later on in the definitive care of a child with

a proven C-spine injury (for instance, during surgery). If a collar is used it should be a good fit (size, adequate positioning).

B – Breathing and ventilation

Evaluate the effectiveness of breathing and ventilation after the airway is opened and high-flow oxygen commenced.

If breathing is ineffective, ventilation must be assisted by BMV with 100% oxygen and tracheal intubation if indicated (Table 11.1). Rarely, a surgical airway may be necessary.

If tracheal intubation is required any neck stabilisation devices must be removed and manual in-line stabilisation maintained during the intubation; a skilled operator is required.

Table 11.1 Indications for intubation and assisted ventilation

- Inadequate oxygenation by bag-mask ventilation
- Prolonged or controlled ventilation required
- Glasgow coma score < 8 or 'P' or 'U' on AVPU score
- Respiratory failure (hypoventilation and/or hypoxia despite 100% oxygen)
- Flail chest, severe facial injuries, or head injury with seizures
- Inhalation injury with burns around the mouth or rest of the face, carboneous sputum or a hoarse voice
- Respiratory arrest

The oral route is preferred for tracheal intubation as the nasotracheal route can lead to neck extension (worsening cervical spine injury), damage to adenoid tissue (with associated haemorrhage) and, in the case of basilar skull fracture, direct damage to the brain.

Emergency anaesthesia for tracheal intubation with cricoid pressure should be considered as the stomach may be full. If cricoid pressure impedes ventilation or intubation however, it should be removed (Chapter 4). Correct tube placement must be confirmed with end-tidal CO_2 and a chest X-ray (should lie between T2 and T3).

Hyperventilation

This should not be performed in children with head injuries as cerebral vasoconstriction induced by hypocapnia aggravates brain ischaemic injuries. The $PaCO_2$ in children with traumatic brain injury (TBI) should be maintained in the lower normal range (4.5–5 kPa).

Gastric distension

Significant gastric distension can occur with swallowed air and BMV. This impairs diaphragmatic movements and affects ventilation. Gastric distension increases the risk of vomiting and aspiration of the stomach contents. A gastric tube should be inserted following intubation. The oral route is preferred in cases of craniofacial trauma (owing to the risk of maxillofacial or basilar skull fractures). The position of the gastric tube must be checked after insertion.

C – Circulation and haemorrhage control

The assessment of cardiovascular status and the restoration of normal circulating volume and hemostasis are key elements of managing a child with haemorrhagic shock; hence two routes of vascular access must be secured in children who have suffered severe trauma. At the same time, blood samples for cross-match, blood gas analysis and laboratory studies must be taken. Some centres also have access to near-patient haemostatic testing which can aid in the management of any coagulopathy. Personal protective equipment should be worn (e.g. gloves, protective clothing, visor/goggles).

Blood loss is the commonest cause of shock in injured children. Blood loss can be visible (i.e. external) or hidden (i.e. internal). Children with burns lose fluids from the burned surface.

Traumatic haemorrhage

Any obvious exsanguinating blood loss from a blood vessel must be controlled by direct pressure, using a thin layer of gauze, even when the amount lost seems small. This is because there may initially be protective vasoconstriction. Haemostatic forceps and tourniquets should not be used except in cases of uncontrolled haemorrhage from traumatic amputation.

Open fractures can cause large quantities of blood to be lost. Splinting of limb fractures (re-establishing normal anatomical position) reduces blood loss, pain and tissue damage.

Pelvic fractures or major long bone closed fractures may also be associated with soft tissue damage and the extravasation of blood. Such injuries when isolated, do not generally lead to hypovolaemic shock in children. In adolescents, when a significant bleeding is suspected from a pelvic fracture with pelvic ring disruption, a pelvic binder should be applied.

Internal haemorrhage

If hypovolaemia persists despite control of external haemorrhage, and the need for fluid resuscitation persists, internal haemorrhage must be excluded. Intra-thoracic, intra-abdominal, retroperitoneal and pelvic bleeding are the main causes of life-threatening internal haemorrhage in children. Intra-abdominal haemorrhage (e.g. rupture of an organ such as the spleen or the liver or major blood vessels) can present with peritonism, abdominal distension (which does not decompress with a gastric tube) and signs of circulatory failure.

Intra-abdominal bleeding, however, may show few signs, hence there must be a high index of suspicion, especially if there is a history of abdominal trauma.

An early focused thoracic and abdominal ultrasound scan may detect free fluid, however a negative ultrasound examination does not rule out severe internal bleeding in children. Children with significant free fluid and continuing haemodynamic instability might need immediate surgical intervention. The gold standard to detect internal bleeding remains contrast-enhanced CT scan (although this has to be balanced against the risk of radiation exposure).

Closed head trauma is not associated with hypovolaemia and another source of bleeding must be sought if hypovolaemic shock is present in a child with head injuries. The exception to this is an acute extradural haemorrhage in the newborn.

Evaluation of blood loss

> - The total circulating blood volume in children is around 70 mL kg^{-1} (depending on age).
> - A decrease in blood pressure is a late sign (often >40% of total blood volume is already lost), and therefore not very useful to initiate or guide treatment.

Evaluation of blood loss (and category of hypovolaemic shock) depends on assessment of respiratory rate, volume of the peripheral pulses, peripheral perfusion (capillary refill time and skin temperature), level of consciousness and BP.

The child should be reassessed repeatedly as there may be rapid alterations in the circulatory status, such as the development of internal haemorrhage (e.g. intra-abdominal bleeding). Response to treatment must also be assessed to see if further interventions are required.

Vascular access

The mainstay of treatment for hypovolaemic shock is intravascular fluid replacement. Circulatory access is usually gained most quickly by the insertion of either two peripheral, short, wide-bore cannulae or by two IO needles (ensuring no IO lines are placed distally to fracture sites (Chapter 5)).

Treatment of hypovolaemic shock

The patient is initially given a 10 mL kg^{-1} bolus of crystalloid which should preferably be warmed to prevent the worsening of hypothermia. Monitoring of the clinical response to each fluid bolus is essential to guide therapy. A further 10 mL kg^{-1} of crystalloid may be administered if there is an inadequate or no response to the initial fluid bolus. Local protocols will dictate the early use of blood products and protocols for massive transfusion will clarify the ratio of packed red cells to fresh frozen plasma, cryoprecipitate and platelets (e.g. The Association of Anaesthetists of Great Britain and Ireland (AAGBI) guideline recommends 1:1 PRBC and FFP with cryoprecipitate and platelets adjusted according to blood results). In all children with massive haemorrhage tranexamic acid should be administered as an initial bolus and then as an infusion for eight hours provided it is started within three hours of injury.

> **Laboratory parameters to aim for:**
>
> - Normal base deficit and lactate level – a trend in base deficit and lactate help monitor the progress of the patient.
>
> - Haemoglobin level 70–90 g L^{-1}
>
> - Platelet count > 100 x 10^9 L^{-1}
>
> - Normal coagulation testing, including fibringogen
>
> - Normal ionised calcium
>
> - Thromboelastography/thromboelastometry (if available)

Intra-abdominal bleeding may be managed conservatively or by angiographic embolisation. Surgery is usually avoided if at all possible. An experienced surgeon will be needed to decide whether operative intervention is necessary to stop internal bleeding. Damage control surgery should focus on bleeding control and brain protection.

D – Disability

The child's disability is determined from his level of consciousness according to the AVPU scale, posture and examination of the pupils for size, symmetry and response to light.

AVPU relates the response (level of consciousness) of the child to a stimulus as follows:

- **A** for ALERT

- **V** for VOICE

- **P** for PAIN

- **U** for UNRESPONSIVE to painful stimulus

An AVPU score of P (i.e. response to pain) is equivalent to a score of eight on the Glasgow coma score when protective gag reflexes are lost. There is, therefore, a risk of aspiration of the stomach contents at this level of consciousness and tracheal intubation must be considered to protect the airway.

The pupils must be examined for size and direct response to light. A unilateral dilated pupil in association with head injury may indicate an intracranial bleed on the same side or raised intracranial pressure and requires urgent neurological referral. Any focal/lateralising signs should be recorded together with the child's posture: arms flexed towards the trunk represents decorticate abnormality, whereas if the child's arms are extended, this may indicate

decerebrate pathology. Both of these postures are worrying and may indicate raised intracranial pressure; the underlying cause must be sought and treated.

The child's vital signs and neurological status must be recorded on a regular basis and the results interpreted in the context of the child's clinical state.

The goal in the primary survey is to diagnose severe head injury, which may require urgent neurosurgical intervention, and/or may determine the need for specific intensive care techniques.

E – Exposure

The child's clothes should be removed in an appropriate manner so that any injuries can be seen in the secondary survey.

As the child has a large body surface to weight ratio, heat loss occurs relatively quickly and he should be covered between examinations and interventions. Warming devices (e.g. overhead radiant heaters, warming blankets, and fluid warmers) should be used to keep the child warm. Marked hypothermia can be deleterious, especially in hypovolaemic shock.

Secondary survey

The secondary survey is a full examination to detect any occult injury. The child should be told what is happening even if he appears to be unconscious. The need for full exposure should be made clear but the child's dignity must be maintained. Further information about the mechanism of injury and forces impacted should be sought.

The secondary survey should only start when all immediate life-threatening injuries have been treated. The vital signs relating to AcBCDE should be regularly assessed during and after the secondary survey; deterioration in the child's clinical signs requires the primary and then the secondary survey to be repeated, stopping to deal with any abnormal clinical features as they are found. In the pre-hospital setting, examination should be limited to the primary survey to exclude life-threatening injuries before and during transportation to the hospital.

As soon as possible, if not performed earlier, blood testing should be performed for blood typing and cross-matching, baseline biochemistry, coagulation and cell count, blood gas analysis and lactate.

X-rays

Routine radiological investigations are carried out at the end of the primary survey, namely:

- chest

- pelvis

- cervical spine.

X-ray of any limb injury must wait until the child is stable and the secondary survey has been completed. These X-rays of the limbs should have an anterior-posterior view as well as lateral view so as not to miss any fractures. Many centres offer swift access to trauma CT scanning for severely injured children instead, but this needs to be balanced with risks of radiation exposure.

History

A short history informs the management of the child and can be remembered by the acronym AMPLE (Table 11.2).

Table 11.2 AMPLE for history taking in secondary survey
A   **Allergy**
M   **Medication**
P   **Past medical history**
L   **Last meal**
E   **Environment (history of accident, mechanism of injury**

Allergy: Allergies must be recorded especially to drugs that may be used (e.g. penicillin).

Medications: Details of current medications (e.g. if the child has a chronic illness such as epilepsy, diabetes or asthma) are important because the drugs used in these conditions may have an impact on the child's management.

Past medical history: The child's past medical history may explain some of the physical signs such as cerebral palsy, although injury must still be excluded.

Last meal: The closer the injury to the time of the last meal the greater the risk of vomiting and potential aspiration; cricoid pressure may be required to protect the airway during intubation (Chapter 4).

Environment: Asking about environment/events gives information about the energy involved in the injury and potential clinical consequences.

Emergency treatment

Emergency treatments for abnormalities found in the secondary survey must be identified and managed as soon as possible after life-threatening injuries are treated.

Analgesia and sedation

This is an essential part of the management of the injured child and should not be delayed. This is usually managed with intravenous or intranasal opiods. Beware of hypoxia, hypovolaemia or hypoglycaemia which can cause symptoms such as aggression or altered level of consciousness.

Definitive care

Definitive care is the final part of the structured approach to trauma. Good note-taking and appropriate referral are essential in providing optimum treatment. These children are frequently transferred to specialist centres and detailed, accurate notes are essential for continuity of care.

Transfer

The transferring team should contact the receiving hospital about the clinical state of the child giving details of suspected injuries, AMPLE, and any procedures or treatments which have been carried out.

The expected time of arrival and the need for additional specialists must be communicated early to ensure their availability. The transferring team must be able to deal with any problem arising during transportation (e.g. deteriorating airway, inadequate ventilation or circulatory problems). External haemorrhage must be controlled before and during transfer and there must be secure intravenous or intraosseous access. The AcBCDE parameters must be evaluated and monitored throughout. When indicated, the transfer should be instigated without delay particularly when a neurosurgical emergency has been identified. Unnecessary examinations and treatments should be avoided, providing the child can be safely transported without deteriorating en route (Chapter 9).

Traumatic brain injury (TBI)

Brain injuries are responsible for 70% of deaths in the first 48 h following paediatric trauma.

Assessment

- history of injury (mechanism of injury, loss of consciousness, headache, vomiting, amnesia, seizures)

- general assessment (AcBCDE), bruises, lacerations, fractures, bleeding from ears and nose or focal neurological pathology

- AcBCDE reassessment should be carried out on a regular basis.

Treatment

Primary brain damage occurs at the time of the trauma and is generally irreversible. Aggressive treatment must be given to prevent secondary brain damage, which may be due to:

- Hypoxia from hypoventilation, airway obstruction, pulmonary contusion, aspiration or seizures (with or without hypoglycaemia).

- Ischaemia which is associated with hypotension, focal/generalised cerebral oedema, extradural/subdural haematoma.

Hypoxia should be ameliorated by administration of 100% oxygen and, if indicated, BMV. Tracheal intubation may be necessary. The underlying cause of hypoxia must also be treated (e.g. pneumothorax).

Secondary brain damage can also be minimised by avoiding systemic hypotension and by treating raised intracranial pressure. Both hypoglycaemia and hyperglycaemia can also worsen the outcome, therefore, ensure careful bedside blood glucose monitoring.

Avoid hypotension and hypoxia in the management of patients with TBI.

Raised intracranial pressure

Raised intracranial pressure (RICP) (e.g. from cerebral oedema), can lead to herniation of the brain through the foramen magnum causing death as the skull has limited ability to expand. It should be identified (ideally prevented) and treated rapidly. It is clinically indicated by depression of conscious level, abnormal pupil size and the Cushing's triad of elevated systemic BP, bradycardia and 'sighing' respirations. Later signs may include decerebrate and or decorticate posturing.

Steps to diminish the likelihood of RICP:

1. The internal jugular veins should not be cannulated for central venous access, as this hinders venous drainage from the brain.

2. The head and chest can be slightly elevated (15–30°), provided there is no evidence of systemic hypotension, to aid venous drainage. Flexion of the body when achieving elevation should be avoided to protect the spinal cord. In case of hypotension, the patient must be kept flat to optimise systemic arterial BP.

3. Mean arterial pressure must be maintained at or above the normal value for the age to preserve cerebral perfusion pressure.

4. Maintain normoxaemia. Hypoxia, especially when combined with hypoperfusion, will induce secondary brain injury. The impact of hyperoxia is unclear at present and you should aim for normal paO_2 or SpO_2 levels.

5. The $PaCO_2$ should be kept between 4.5–5.0 kPa (i.e. within the normal range). Hyperventilation should only be carried out under careful supervision if there is an acute rise in ICP.

6. Hypertonic saline or mannitol must be given if there is evidence of RICP. Monitoring of serum osmolality and urine output via urinary catheterisation (via the suprapubic route if there is urethral trauma) is essential. In unilateral lesions without evidence of RICP consult a neurosurgical specialist before administering.

---

7. Hyperglycaemia and hypoglycaemia must be avoided.

8. Seizures should be treated with benzodiazepines and antiepileptic medication as required.

9. Provide adequate analgesia and sedation. Pain and stress increase cerebral metabolic demands therefore leading to increased cerebral blood flow and ultimately a further increase in ICP.

Hypovolaemic shock in brain injuries

Isolated closed head injuries do not usually cause hypovolaemic shock and internal haemorrhage must be considered as a cause. Other causes such as intrathoracic or intra-abdominal trauma, pelvic and long bone fractures must be ruled out. Scalp lacerations, and in certain cases acute extradural haemorrhage in the newborn, can lead to a significant blood loss so the scalp must be carefully inspected.

The most common cause of death in trauma is hypovolaemic shock. Fluid and blood transfusions, when indicated, are essential to maintain adequate cerebral blood flow to prevent worsening of any co-existing brain injury.

Investigations of cerebral lesions

Haemodynamically stable patients can have CT scans of the brain. However, resuscitation equipment and a resuscitation team must be on hand as the seemingly stabilised patient can suddenly deteriorate.

A CT scan may demonstrate treatable conditions such as:

- skull fractures (compound and depressed, including basilar skull fractures associated with 0.4–5% risk infection)

- intracranial haemorrhages (extradural haematoma, subdural haematoma, cerebral contusions and subarachnoid haemorrhage)

- midline shift of white and grey matter

- signs of cerebral oedema and RICP (absent sulci, slit-like cerebral ventricles).

Extradural haematoma

Extradural haematomas are life-threatening emergencies requiring extremely urgent drainage by a neurosurgeon. A rapidly expanding extradural haematoma can cause cerebral herniation so time is of the essence even if the child is clinically unstable.

Systemic arterial hypertension

Systemic hypertension associated with bradycardia and irregular respiration (Cushing's triad) suggests RICP. The systemic hypertension should not be treated with antihypertensive agents but RICP should be managed appropriately.

Hyperglycaemia

Hyperglycaemia aggravates ischaemic cerebral lesions. Administration of glucose-containing solutions must be avoided during resuscitation, unless given to treat documented hypoglycaemia. Blood sugar levels must be monitored.

Chest trauma (primary survey)

Life-threatening conditions such as tension pneumothorax, massive haemothorax, flail chest and cardiac tamponade can be identified and treated during the primary survey. If the child deteriorates during the secondary survey, or later due to one of these conditions, the primary survey must be repeated.

Pneumothorax

Pneumothorax means that there is air, between the lung and the internal thoracic wall, which compresses the lung and impedes ventilation. There are three mains types – simple, tension and open. Respiratory failure can be caused by all three.

All forms of pneumothorax can be diagnosed clinically.

Simple pneumothorax

This represents a limited air leak into the pleural space, which causes the lung to collapse without there being significant haemodynamic signs.

A small simple pneumothorax may only be identified on secondary survey and chest X-ray. It may be managed conservatively provided there is continuous monitoring of the child's physiological parameters to ensure there is no deterioration in the clinical condition. Immediate chest drainage is required if the child requires ventilation. This is because the simple pneumothorax is sometimes not discovered prior to intubation. The pressures involved in ventilation can convert a simple pneumothorax to a tension pneumothorax, which can lead to the patient becoming difficult to ventilate – this should be always considered.

Tension pneumothorax

When air is forced into the pleural cavity (a limited space) without means of escape, it accumulates and comes under pressure. This pressure can displace the mediastinum to the opposite side of the chest causing compression of the great vessels, so interfering with venous return, causing obstructive shock with a concomitant fall in systemic BP. The jugular venous pressure is raised if there is no associated hypovolaemia.

Signs:

- hypoxia

- absent/decreased breath sounds on affected side

- neck vein distension

- tracheal deviation away from the side of the tension pneumothorax.

Treatment:

1. Airway opening.

2. Oxygen (100%) by face mask or BMV.

3. Needle thoracocentesis – the insertion of a cannula into the second intercostal space in the mid-clavicular line on the side of the tension pneumothorax (Figure 11.2). When the needle of the cannula is removed, a hiss of escaping air may be heard as the pressure within the pleural space is released. The cannula is left to vent the air if the patient is ventilated but if spontaneously breathing it will need to be capped and be aspirated intermittently until a chest drain is placed.

4. Chest drain insertion should be undertaken as soon as possible, provided it doesn't delay progressing the assessment and management of the patient.

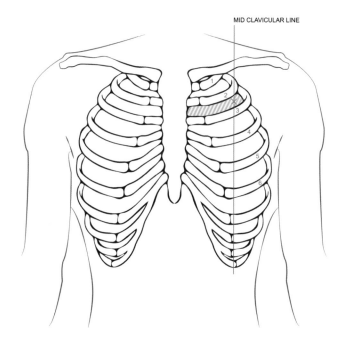

Figure 11.2 Landmark for needle thoracocentesis (X)

If the child deteriorates at any stage following the needle thoracocentesis, air may have reaccumulated, reforming the tension pneumothorax. This may be due to the cannula kinking. Needle thoracocentesis must be repeated and a chest drain inserted as soon as possible.

Open pneumothorax

Open pneumothorax results from a penetrating chest wound and makes a sucking noise. When the child breathes in, a negative intrathoracic pressure is generated (which normally draws air into the lungs with each inspiration) and air rushes in through the wound into the pleural space. This then leads to inefficient ventilation and displacement of the mediastinum with each breath causing cardiovascular instability. If the open chest wound is obstructed, therefore causing a one-way valve effect, a tension pneumothorax can also develop.

- penetrating chest wound (examine front and back)

- audible air passage through the wound

- decreased chest wall movement on affected side

- decreased breath sounds on affected side

- increased percussion noted on affected side

- a tension pneumothorax can develop from an open pneumothorax.

Treatment:

1. Airway opening.

2. Oxygen (100%) by face mask or BMV.

3. Close the defect with a chest seal dressing (e.g. Russel or Asherman), which will seal the wound and allow entrapped air to escape through a valve. These are more effective than the previously used occlusive dressing taped down on three sides.

4. Chest drain insertion on the same side as the pneumothorax but in an area away from the wound.

If a tension pneumothorax is present, treat accordingly. If positive pressure ventilation is required a chest drain must be sited as soon as possible.

Massive haemothorax

This is due to blood accumulating in the thoracic cavity as a result of a pulmonary parenchymal injury associated with pulmonary vessels or chest wall injuries. A haemothorax may contain a significant proportion of a child's total circulatory blood volume.

Signs:

- hypoxia

- hypovolaemic shock

- decreased chest wall movements on affected side

- decreased breath sounds on affected side

- decreased percussion noted on affected side

- neck veins may be flat, not full or distended.

Treatment:

1. Airway opening.

2. Oxygen (100%) by face mask or BMV.

3. Vascular access with two large bore intravenous cannulae or intraosseous needles.

4. Fluid infusion (10 mL kg^{-1}) bolus(es). Blood should be used as soon as it is available.

5. Insertion of chest drain.

As blood loss can be rapid via the chest drain, fluid replacement must be available and circulatory access secured before its insertion. Temporary clamping of the chest drain and an urgent thoracotomy may be required if the initial blood drainage is > 20 mL kg^{-1}, with persistent loss requiring continuing blood transfusion.

Flail chest

Flail chest is where two or more ribs are broken in two or more places so that they are not connected to the rest of the rib cage and do not move in conjunction with it on expiration and inspiration. Hypoventilation may occur, and respiratory failure can develop as a result of pain and severe pulmonary contusions that usually accompanies a flail chest. This is very uncommon in childhood owing to the child's increased chest wall elasticity.

Cardiac tamponade

Cardiac tamponade generally results from penetrating rather than blunt injuries. Therefore, cardiac tamponade is not often seen in paediatric trauma. The heart is pierced and blood fills the pericardial sac. This limits the space for cardiac contraction causing obstructive shock. Cardiac tamponade requires emergency thoracotomy. Pericardiocentesis might be attempted if immediate thoracotomy is not available. The procedure should be guided by ultrasound and a pericardial drain should be inserted.

Chest trauma (secondary survey)

Rib fractures

Rib injuries are always significant as they suggest considerable trauma in children. Underlying chest and abdominal injuries must be suspected.

Upper rib (1–3) and clavicle fractures suggest injury to the major vessels, the mediastinum, and the bronchus. Fractures of the middle ribs (4–9) are associated with pulmonary contusion and haemothorax, while the lower ribs (10–12) are linked to liver and splenic injuries.

Ensure analgesia and examination for underlying damage, such as thoracic or abdominal injury.

Pulmonary contusion

Pulmonary contusion is common in childhood, even in the absence of fractures. It results from the disruption of pulmonary capillaries and the filling of the alveoli with blood, thus leading to hypoxia. Treatment is based on oxygenation, and mechanical ventilation may be required. Ensure analgesia and respiratory physiotherapy is important and useful.

Tracheobronchial tree injuries

Tracheobronchial tree ruptures are associated with a pneumothorax or haemothorax with subcutaneous emphysema. They should be considered in the presence of a persistent large air leak after insertion of a chest drain.

Great vessel injuries

Great vessel injuries are rapidly fatal, except if the leak is contained within the vessel wall. The child may present with shock, and a high index of suspicion should be triggered by a widened mediastinum on the chest X-ray. Diagnosis is confirmed by CT-angiography and urgent surgical treatment is required.

Traumatic diaphragmatic hernia

A traumatic diaphragmatic hernia occurs more often following abdominal trauma, and is more common on the left side. Diagnosis can be made from hearing bowel sounds on chest auscultation and seeing bowel within the chest cavity on chest X-ray. Often the child will refuse to lie down. These injuries may occur with lap seat belts and treatment is surgical repair.

Abdominal trauma

The ability to determine the presence of intra-abdominal bleeding is poor without accompanying investigation; note that abdominal haemorrhage is often associated with blunt trauma. If there is any suggestive history or sign, such as distension or contusions on the abdominal wall, surgical opinion and investigations are urgently required (e.g. abdominal ultrasonography) to rule out free intraperitoneal fluid.

Signs:

- abdominal wall contusion

- abdominal wall bruising, lacerations or penetrating wounds

- abdominal distension

- abdominal or shoulder tip pain

- peritoneal irritation or peritonitis

- hypovolaemic shock unresponsive to fluid resuscitation.

Gentle examination of the abdomen should be carried out as it may reveal an area of tenderness and rigidity suggestive of intra-abdominal haemorrhage. It is important to note, however, that inspection, palpation, percussion and auscultation may not detect intra-abdominal bleeding. Gastric and urinary bladder drainage may help in the assessment by decompressing the abdomen. Vaginal examination should only be performed by a clinician with expertise in gynaecological trauma and only if indicated. The external urethral meatus of the penis should be examined for blood as well as the scrotum for any collection of blood. The rectal examination should only be carried out once during the secondary survey, ideally by the surgeon responsible for deciding if operative treatment is required.

Investigations:

- Blood tests: full blood count, cross-match, urea, electrolytes, amylase, bedside estimation of blood glucose, and clotting profiles.

- X-rays: of the three secondary survey X-rays, the chest and pelvic ones may suggest intra-abdominal injury (e.g. free gas under the diaphragm), soft tissue swelling and incorrect location of the gastric tube (as in traumatic diaphragmatic hernia).

- Ultrasound may show the presence of free fluid within the abdominal cavity; laceration of intra-abdominal organs such as the liver or spleen.

- Diagnostic peritoneal lavage should not be performed.

- CT scan of the abdomen is the imaging investigation of choice for every severely injured child; however, a CT scan should only be performed if the child is sufficiently haemodynamically stable. Any child with significant injury going to the CT scan must be escorted by a medical team competent in performing paediatric resuscitation and appropriate equipment and drugs must be available. In children with less severe presumed injuries (less severe trauma mechanism) the decision to do an abdominal CT scan must be balanced against the risks of radiation exposure.

Treatment:

Most children with visceral injury are managed non-surgically but on a site where there is a supervising experienced surgeon and team on-site, ready to operate should the child deteriorate. Indications for operative intervention include penetrating injury, perforated bowel, refractory hypovolaemic shock (i.e. unresponsive to fluid resuscitation).

Skeletal trauma

Skeletal trauma is rarely life-threatening; its appearance, however, must not detract from adherence to AcBCDE steps of managing an injured child.

The few life-threatening conditions in skeletal trauma which are treated in the primary and secondary survey include:

1. Crush injury of the abdomen and pelvis.

2. Traumatic amputation of an extremity, either partial or complete.

3. Massive long bone open fracture.

Additionally, neurovascular injuries and compartment syndrome should be identified early as they can become limb threatening.

Crush injury of the abdomen and pelvis

Crush injury of the abdomen and pelvis is associated with hypovolaemic shock which remains resistant to fluid resuscitation until the pelvic disruption is stabilised and injured vessels are occluded. This is initially achieved with a pelvic binder and then by using an external pelvic fixator, radiological intervention or by operative means. In either case, urgent surgical management is required. Limit the number of examinations of pelvic stability as this may increase bleeding. Never insert a urinary catheter unless urethral injury has been ruled out.

Traumatic amputation

In complete amputation, blood loss is usually limited owing to the transected blood vessels going into spasm for a limited time. In partial amputation there may be considerable blood loss as blood vessel spasm may not occur; urgent management is needed. The child may need to be treated for hypovolaemic shock.

Direct pressure should be applied to the bleeding vessels with a haemostatic dressing or gauze. A tourniquet should be placed proximally on a limb to help stop torrential bleeding – this is only a short-term measure to provide time to definitive surgical management to stop the bleeding.

An amputated limb should be isolated in a sterile bag and then kept cool (avoiding direct contact with any ice being used as a coolant) until a surgical opinion about the feasibility of surgical re-attachment is obtained.

Open long bone fractures

This is usually obvious and needs immediate treatment if there is associated exsanguinating haemorrhage; direct pressure should be applied to the bleeding vessels with a haemostatic dressing or gauze. Splinting the limb so that the correct anatomical position is achieved will help to reduce blood loss, pain, tissue damage and the risk of compartment syndrome. Expert orthopaedic help is needed to manage this condition. The child may be in hypovolaemic shock and should be treated for this.

Limbs

The extremities should be inspected for bruising, swelling, deformity, laceration, and any evidence of open fractures. Gentle palpation should be undertaken to establish any areas of tenderness and to evaluate the surface temperature and capillary refill time.

The neurovascular status of the limb, especially distal to injury, must be recorded and acted upon (e.g. the absence of pulses distal to a supracondylar fracture can be limb-threatening unless managed urgently).

Assessment of the vascular status of the limb relies on determining:

- The presence and quality of peripheral pulses distal to the injury.

- Capillary refill time and skin temperature gradient compared with the rest of the body.

- Sensory and motor function (i.e. neurological status of the limb)

- A large bruise or haematoma is suggestive of vascular injury, particularly if it continues to increase in size.

Emergency treatment of vascular limb injury:

1. Fluid resuscitation with 10 mL kg^{-1} bolus(es) with haemostasis of obvious bleeding. Consider administering blood products early to prevent a dilutional anaemia.

2. Pain relief.

3. Alignment and immobilisation by splintage (if pain increases after immobilisation, then ischaemic injury and/or compartment syndrome must be excluded).

Compartment syndrome

This occurs when the interstitial pressure is higher than the capillary tissue pressure in the fascial compartment, and local muscle ischaemia results. It may occur, for example, in a circumferential burn of the upper arm. The burn impedes venous blood drainage out of the limb (which has a maximum venous BP of 10–15 mmHg). However, the systemic arterial flow into the arm continues as the systemic BP is much higher. There is a 'damming-up' of blood within the muscle of the forearm and the increasing pressure is transmitted to the tissues via the capillary bed, leading to muscle ischaemia and cellular necrosis.

Signs:

- pain accentuated by passive muscle stretch

- decreased sensation

- swelling

- muscle weakness.

Distal pulses only disappear when the intracompartmental pressure rises above arterial BP. Initial treatment is the releasing of any constrictions. Surgical intervention may be required (i.e. fasciotomies to try to save the limb).

Cervical spine injury

Compared to an adult a child has a relatively large head, immature vertebral bodies (with less tensile strength) through which the spinal cord travels, strong elastic intervertebral ligaments, flexible joint capsules and easily compressible soft tissue in the neck.

As these structures are pliable, injury to the cervical spinal cord may occur without radiographic abnormality being seen (SCIWORA). This holds true for the rest of the spine.

Although spinal cord injury is uncommon, the cervical spine must be immobilised along with the rest of the spine until spinal cord injury can be clinically excluded by neurological examination.

Signs:

- severe multiple injuries

- significant trauma to the head, neck and back

- any trauma associated with high deceleration forces such as high velocity traffic accidents

- falls from heights.

Conscious children may complain of pain in the affected vertebra(e).

In the assessment, the six 'Ps' should be evaluated:

- Pain

- Position

- Paralysis

- Paresthaesia

- Priapism

- Ptosis (for upper cervical lesions).

If pain, tenderness or swelling located to the spinal area are present, even in the absence of neurological signs, spinal injury must be ruled out. Magnetic resonance imaging is a useful diagnostic tool.

Treatment:

1. Treatment is based on the AcBCDE process. Airway obstruction is common in such patients and a jaw thrust manoeuvre should be carried out, avoiding movement of the cervical spine.

2. Cervical immobilisation using manual in-line stabilisation or head blocks with two points of attachment to prevent neck movement must be employed.

3. Ventilation should be assisted if there is respiratory failure or risk to the airway. Tracheal intubation is a skilled technique and should be carried out by an experienced intubator. It requires in-line cervical spine immobilisation by an assistant.

Burns

Burns (thermal injuries) are described by:

Depth

- First degree (superficial) burns have generalised erythema, as seen in sunburn.

- Second degree (partial thickness) burns show blistering of skin, but this remains pink or slightly mottled. Both first and second degree burns are painful.

- Third degree (full thickness) burns appear white or charred and as the pain receptors in the deep dermis have been ablated, they are painless.

Location burns to the face, hands, feet and perineum are always considered serious; they have specific management considerations regardless of their depth.

Body surface area (BSA) the involved area should be calculated from a paediatric burns chart. These charts show the age-related change in percentage BSA of the head, limbs, trunk and body. A useful method of quickly determining BSA is to measure the area of the child's palm with the fingers spread out as this is 1% BSA. The 'rule of nines' cannot be applied to a child younger than 14 years. Local burns surgeons should be involved in the development of management protocols.

Airway

The upper airway may be compromised owing to injury from burns or chemical irritants from noxious agents. As oedema quickly follows, the airway may deteriorate rapidly and even the suspicion of potential airway compromise should prompt immediate consideration of tracheal intubation; delay may make intubation impossible. Worrying features include facial burns, singed eyebrows or carbon stained sputum. The use of low pressure cuffed tubes is preferable in view of expected problems with mechanical ventilation.

Breathing

In severe cases, there may be circumferential burns to the thorax which limits its movement. Releasing incisions may be required to reduce the constricting effect of the burns (escharotomies). Particles inhaled during fire may contribute to respiratory distress and must be removed by suction after intubation or bronchoscopy. Oxygen 100% should be administered to all cases of severe burns as there maybe carbon monoxide poisoning.

Circulation

Fluid resuscitation (10 mL kg^{-1} of isotonic fluid) is necessary if there are signs of shock with careful reassessment after each bolus.

Children with burns of 10% or more require extra fluid, in addition to daily maintenance requirements using the formula:

$$\boxed{\text{BSA \% x Bodyweight (kg) x 4 mL day}^{-1}}$$

Careful fluid-balance monitoring is necessary in the management of burned children including urine output. The time for the additional fluid requirement starts at the time that the burn occurred.

Pain relief

Any child with anything other than a minor burn should be given morphine, IV or IO (0.1 mg kg^{-1}) titrated to their needs. Initial routes of administration of opioids such as diamorphine or fentanyl can be given via the intranasal route until such time as an intravascular route is secured.

Wound Care

Wound care should be started as soon as possible to avoid infection. Hypothermia should be avoided. The child's tetanus status should be determined to identify if a tetanus booster is required.

Drowning

Drowning causes respiratory impairment from immersion (at least face and upper airway covered) or submersion (all the body) in water or another fluid. The most common and detrimental consequence of drowning is hypoxia. The duration of hypoxia is the critical factor in determining outcome.

Terms such as dry or wet drowning, near-drowning or silent drowning should not be used.

Safety

Personal safety is always a priority. Attempt to save the child without entry into the water. Try to reach the child with a rescue aid (e.g. stick, clothing), throwing a rope or a buoyant rescue aid or using a boat. If entry into water is essential, a floating device (e.g. buoyant rescue aid) should be used.

The child should be removed from the water by the fastest and safest means available. Remove the victim from the water in a horizontal position to avoid post-drowning hypotension and cardiovascular collapse if possible.

Airway

Cervical spine injury is rare and c-spine immobilisation is difficult to perform in the water. Cervical spine immobilisation is therefore not indicated unless severe injury is likely (e.g. diving, waterslide use). Open the airway by jaw thrust if possible.

Breathing

In-water rescue breathing should be performed only if the rescuer is trained to do so. Otherwise, rescue breathing must be started when out of the water (or in shallow water) if there is no spontaneous breathing after opening the airway.

Circulation

If there are no signs of life or a central pulse, start chest compressions.

Advanced life support in drowning

1. Airway and breathing.

2. High-flow oxygen should be given during initial assessment of the spontaneously breathing child.

3. Non-invasive ventilation or CPAP may also be applied if hypoxia persists.

4. Early tracheal intubation and ventilation should be considered in children who are not responding to these measures or have a reduced level of consciousness.

5. Assess circulation for hypovolaemic shock and give bolus of fluid as indicated but avoid fluid overload.

Hypothermia

Actively rewarm the child until a core temperature of 32–34°C is achieved. The body temperature should be carefully monitored during subsequent period of intensive care.

Non-accidental injury

Non-accidental injury may present as a physical injury. This is only one form of child abuse; others include nutritional deprivation, neglect, emotional or sexual abuse and deliberate poisoning. There may be a history of domestic violence. Healthcare professionals must pay attention to any clues, such as:

- The history being incompatible with the clinical findings, frequently changing, being inconsistent with the child's motor development or improbably complex.

- The interval between time of injury and presentation at the hospital being inexplicably long.

- The trauma is repetitive (e.g. many bruises in different locations).

- The parental answer being inappropriate (unduly aggressive, apparently unconcerned or over-anxious).

- Histories told by parents or carers are divergent.

Injuries must be managed according to the AcBCDE principles with the involvement of child protection experts such as the paediatric team. The child should be protected against possible repetition of injury. The safety of other siblings must also be considered. The case should be managed by a senior clinician, preferably experienced in child protection procedures.

Summary learning

- Trauma is the second highest cause of death in children over 10 years old.
- Treat first what kills first – deal with life threatening problems as they are found (AcBCDE).
- Trauma management requires surgical expertise.
- Secondary survey is a thorough head-to-toe examination, front and back.
- If the child deteriorates, repeat the primary survey.
- Airway patency can be rapidly lost in upper airway burns.
- Drowning children must be removed from water by the fastest and safest means.
- Non-accidental injury must be considered in injured children.

My key take-home messages from this chapter

Welsh systematic child protection group
http://www.core-info.cardiff.ac.uk/

Further reading

American College of Surgeons. Advanced Trauma Life Support Course. 8th ed. Chicago, III: American College of surgeons. 2008.

Pang D, Pollack IF. Spinal cord injury without radiographic abnormalities in children: the SCIWORA syndrome. J Trauma. 1989; 29: 654-664.

Faculty of Clinical Radiology. Paediatric trauma protocols. The Royal College of Radiologists, 2014.

UK trauma care practice.
http://www.trauma.myzen.co.uk/contact.html

Babies born outside the delivery room

Contents

- **Resuscitation of the newborn outside the delivery room**
- **Principles of assessment and management of newborn resuscitation**
- **Algorithm for NLS**
- **Drugs used in newborn resuscitation**
- **Preterm newborns**
- **Discontinuation of resuscitation**

Learning outcomes

To enable you to:

- **Identify the equipment required for newborn resuscitation**
- **Formulate strategies for newborn resuscitation**
- **Undertake assessment of the newborn infant**
- **Identify differences in preterm babies**
- **Think about when to consider discontinuation newborn resuscitation**

The resuscitation of babies at birth is different from the resuscitation of all other age groups as the baby must change, from a being with fluid-filled lungs whose respiratory function is carried out by the placenta to a separate being whose air-filled lungs can successfully take over this function. The majority of newly born babies will establish normal respiration and circulation without help.

Birth outside the delivery room

Ideally, someone trained in newborn resuscitation should be present at all deliveries. However, some babies are born in unexpected places (e.g. emergency departments) and for these situations it is important that clinicians have an understanding of the differences in resuscitating a baby at birth.

Whenever a baby is born unexpectedly there is often great difficulty in keeping it warm, but this is **very important** to avoid both morbidity and mortality. Drying and wrapping, turning up the heating and closing windows and doors are all important in maintaining the body temperature.

Hospitals with emergency departments should have guidelines for resuscitation at birth, summoning help and post-resuscitation transfer of babies born within the department.

Babies born unexpectedly, outside hospital, will be at greater risk of being pre-term and of getting cold. However, the principles of resuscitation are identical to the hospital setting. Transport will need to be discussed according to local guidelines.

Equipment

For many newborn babies, especially those born outside the delivery room, the need for resuscitation cannot be predicted. It is therefore useful to plan for such an eventuality. Equipment, which may be required to resuscitate a newborn baby, is listed in Table 12.1. This will vary between departments; however, most babies can be resuscitated with a flat surface, warmth, knowledge and a way to deliver air or oxygen at a controlled pressure.

Strategy for assessing and resuscitating a baby at birth

Resuscitation is likely to be rapidly successful if begun before the baby has become so anoxic that all potential for respiratory activity has vanished.

Table 12.1 Equipment for newborn resuscitation

- A flat surface
- Source of warmth and dry towels
- A plastic bag or wrap
- A suction system with catheters at least 12 Fr
- Stethoscope and or saturation monitor
- Face masks
- Bag-valve mask or pressure-limiting device
- Source of air and oxygen
- Oropharyngeal airways
- Laryngoscopes with size 0 and 1 blades
- Nasogastric tubes
- Device to clamp cord
- Scissors
- Tracheal tubes sizes 2.5 to 4.0 mm
- Tracheal tube stylet
- Umbilical catheters
- Adhesive tape
- Disposable gloves

Always start by drying and covering the baby to prevent it from getting cold and then proceed as far as is necessary down the following list:

- Call for help
- Start the clock or note the time
- Dry and cover the baby
- Assess the situation
- Airway
- Breathing

- Chest compressions
- (Drugs).

Figure 12.1 Newborn life support algorithm.

Call for help

Ask for help if you expect or encounter any difficulty or if the delivery is outside a labour suite.

Start clock

Start the clock if available, or note the time of birth.

At birth

- There is no need to rush to clamp the cord, particularly if the baby appears well. Unless the baby is clearly in need of immediate resuscitation, wait for at least one minute from the complete delivery of the baby before clamping the cord. Keep the baby warm during this time.

- Dry the baby quickly and effectively. Remove the wet towel and wrap in a fresh dry warm towel. For very small or significantly preterm babies it is better to place the wet baby in a food-grade plastic bag – and then under a radiant heater.

- Assess the baby and decide whether any intervention is going to be needed.

- Clamp and cut the cord.

If the baby is thought to need assistance then this becomes the priority and the cord may need to be clamped in order to deliver that assistance. This is especially likely in deliveries occurring in unexpected areas. When cutting the cord make sure it is securely tied to prevent blood loss.

Keep the baby warm

Dry the baby immediately and then wrap in a dry towel. Babies who become cold (<36.5 °C) are significantly more likely to die. If this is not addressed at the beginning of resuscitation it is often forgotten. Most of the heat loss is caused by the baby being wet and in a draught – hence the need to dry the baby and then to wrap the baby in a dry towel. Babies also have a large surface area to weight ratio; thus heat can be lost very quickly. Ideally, delivery should take place in a warm room, and an overhead heater should be switched on. However, drying effectively and wrapping the baby in a warm dry towel is the most important factor in avoiding hypothermia. A naked wet baby can still become hypothermic despite a warm room and a radiant heater, especially if there is a draught. Make sure that the head is covered as it represents a significant part of the baby's surface area (see pre-term babies, below).

Assessment of the newborn baby

Whilst keeping the baby warm make an initial assessment by assessing:

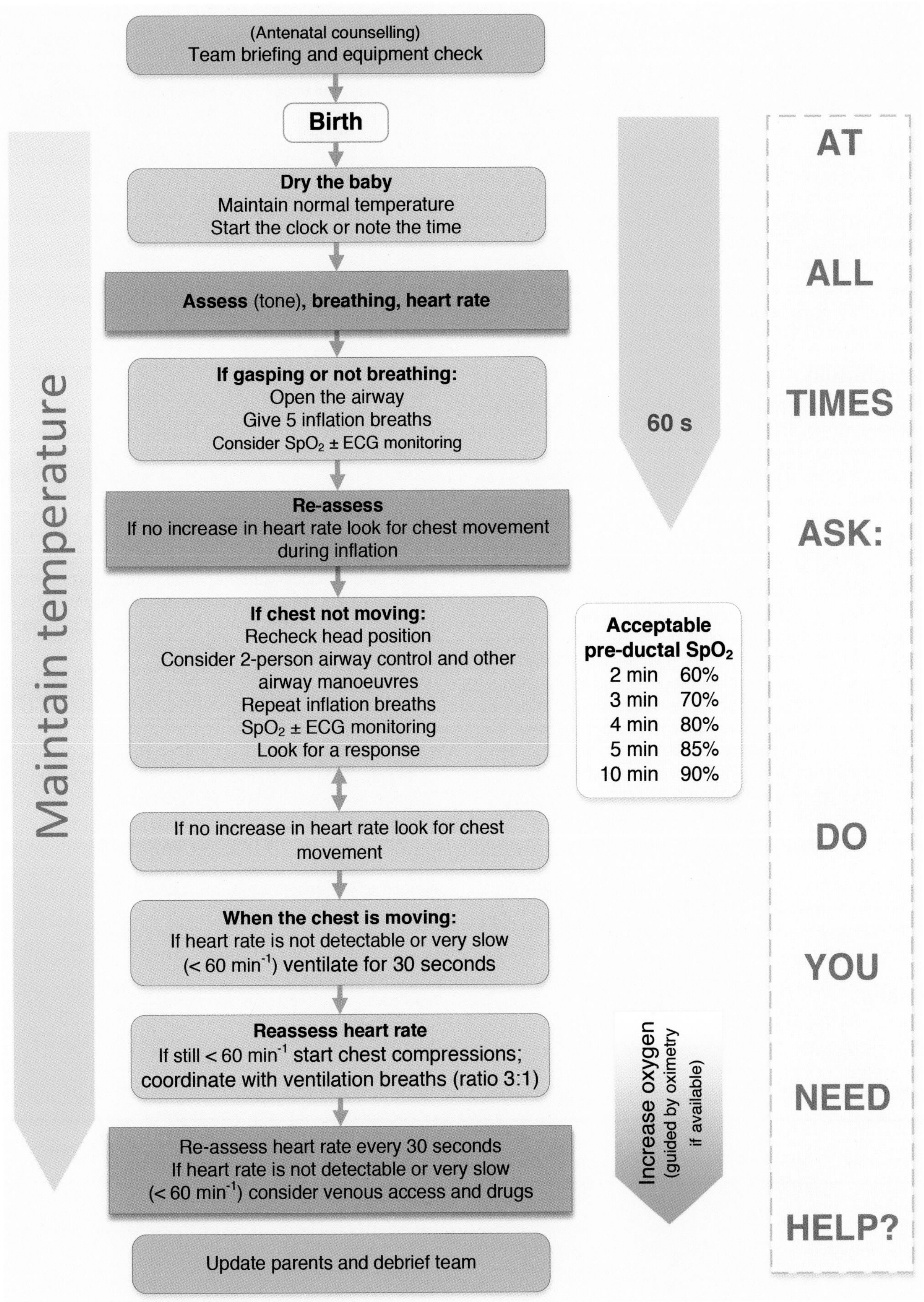

Figure 12.1 Newborn life support algorithm

- Respiration (rate and quality), Airway and Breathing

- Heart rate (e.g. fast, slow, absent)

- Colour (e.g. pink, blue, pale), Circulation

- Tone (e.g. unconscious, apnoeic babies are floppy).

Unlike resuscitation at other ages, it is important to regularly re-assess the newborn and at fairly short intervals of 30 s so that one can judge the success of interventions. This is most true of **heart rate** and **breathing**, which guide further resuscitative efforts. However, a baby who is white and shut down peripherally is more likely to be acidotic and a baby who is floppy (atonic) is likely to be unconscious. Subsequent assessments should focus on breathing and heart rate.

Respiration

Most babies will establish spontaneous regular breathing sufficient to maintain the heart rate above 100 min^{-1} and to improve the skin colour within three minutes of birth. If apnoea or gasping persists after drying, intervention is required.

Heart rate

In the first couple of minutes after birth, auscultating at the cardiac apex or applying an ECG is the best method to assess the heart rate. Palpating peripheral pulses is not practical and cannot be recommended. Palpation of the umbilical pulse can only be relied upon if it is > 100 min^{-1}. A rate less than this should be checked by auscultation if possible or by a saturation monitor using masimo (or similar) technology if available. A saturation monitor applied to the right hand or wrist (i.e. pre-ductal) can give an accurate reading of heart rate and saturations within 90 s of application (see later). An initial assessment of heart rate is vital because an increase in the heart rate will be the first sign of success during resuscitation.

It is usually clear whether the heart rate is very slow (< 60 min^{-1}), slow (60–100 min^{-1}) or fast (> 100 min^{-1}). It is not necessary to count it with complete accuracy. A heart rate below 100 min^{-1} is abnormal.

Colour

Attempting to judge oxygenation by assessing skin colour is unreliable but it is still worth noting the baby's colour at birth as well as when and how it changes. Very pale babies who remain pale after resuscitation may be hypovolaemic as well as acidotic.

If the baby has good tone, a good heart rate and is making good respiratory effort then further help is unlikely to be needed.

Using an oxygen saturation monitor will allow rapid assessment of heart rate and saturation within about 90 s of application. Oxygen saturation levels in healthy babies in the first few minutes of life may be considerably lower than at other times (Table 12.2).

Table 12.2 Time from birth and acceptable preductal percentage value of peripheral oxygen saturation (% SpO$_2$)

Time from birth (min)	Acceptable (25th centile) preductal saturation (% SpO$_2$)
2	60
3	70
4	80
5	85
10	90

This assessment will categorise the baby into one of the three following groups:

1. Regular respirations, heart rate fast (> 100 min^{-1}) pink, good tone. These are healthy babies and they should be kept warm and given to their mothers. The baby will remain warm through skin-to-skin contact with the mother under a cover and may be put to the breast at this stage under supervision.

2. Irregular or inadequate respirations, heart rate slow (< 100 min^{-1}), blue, normal or reduced tone. If gentle stimulation (such as drying) does not induce effective breathing, the airway should be opened and, if necessary, cleared. If the baby responds then no further resuscitation is needed. If there is no response, progress to lung inflation.

3. Apnoeic, heart rate slow (< 100 min^{-1}) or absent, blue or pale, floppy. Open the airway and then inflate the lungs. A reassessment of any heart rate response then directs further resuscitation. Reassess the heart rate and respiration at regular intervals throughout.

Apnoea, low or absent heart rate, pallor and floppiness together suggest terminal apnoea. However, initial management of such babies is unchanged but resuscitation may be prolonged.

After assessment, resuscitation follows:

- Airway

- Breathing

- Circulation

- With the use of drugs in a few selected cases.

Airway

The baby should be positioned with the head in the neutral position (Figure 12.2).

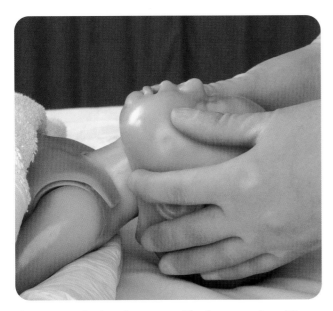

Figure 12.2 The head supported in the neutral position with jaw thrust

The newborn baby's head has a large, often moulded, occiput, which tends to cause the neck to flex when the baby is supine on a flat surface. However, overextension may also collapse the newborn baby's pharyngeal airway, leading to obstruction. A 2 cm folded towel placed under the neck and shoulders may help to maintain the airway in a neutral position and a jaw thrust may be needed to bring the tongue forward and open the airway, especially if the baby is floppy. Although these rarely cause airway obstruction, visible secretions may be removed by gentle suction with a paediatric Yankauer or 12–14 Fr suction catheter. Blind deep pharyngeal suction should not be performed as it may cause vagally induced bradycardia and laryngospasm. Suction, if it is used, should not exceed –150 mmHg (20 kPa). The presence of thick meconium (see below) in a non-vigorous baby is the only indication for considering visualization of the oropharynx and immediate suction.

Meconium aspiration

Meconium-stained liquor (light green tinge) is relatively common and occurs in up to 10% of births. Meconium aspiration is a rare event. Usually occurring in term infants in-utero before delivery.

Breathing (aeration breaths and ventilation)

The first five breaths in term babies should be inflation breaths in order to replace lung fluid in the alveoli with air. These should be 2–3 s sustained breaths using a continuous gas supply, a pressure-limiting device and a mask. Use a transparent, circular soft mask big enough to cover the nose and mouth of the baby. If no such system is available, or you are not familiar with it, then a 500 mL self-inflating bag and a blow-off valve set at 30–40 cm H_2O can be used. This is especially useful if compressed air or oxygen is not available.

The chest may not move during the first 1–3 breaths as fluid is displaced. Adequate ventilation is usually indicated by either a rapidly increasing heart rate or a heart rate that is maintained at > 100 min[-1]. Therefore, reassess the heart rate after delivery of the first five breaths. It is safe to assume the chest has been successfully inflated if the heart rate responds. Once the chest is inflated and the heart rate has increased or the chest has been seen to move, ventilation should be continued at a rate of 30–40 min[-1]. Continue ventilatory support until regular breathing is established. Where possible, start resuscitation of the baby at birth with air. There is now good evidence for this in term babies and oxygen toxicity is a real concern with premature babies. Use of supplemental oxygen should be guided by pulse oximetry with reasonable levels listed and on the algorithm (Table 12.2 and Figure 12.1).

If, despite effective ventilation heart rate remains low or oxygenation (guided by pulse oximetry) remains unacceptable, use of a higher concentration of oxygen should be considered. Note: if only 100% oxygen is available then this should be used and resuscitation should not be delayed. Resuscitation of preterm babies may be initiated using air 30% oxygen.

Circulation

If the heart rate remains slow or absent, despite adequate ventilation for 30 s as shown by chest movement, then chest compressions should be started. Chest compressions will help to move oxygenated blood from the lungs to the heart and coronary arteries.

The most efficient way of delivering chest compressions in the neonate is to encircle the chest with both hands, so that the fingers lie behind the baby and the thumbs overlap on the sternum just below the inter-nipple line (Figure12.3). Compress the chest briskly, by one third of its depth. In newborn babies, perform three compressions for each ventilation breath (3:1 ratio).

The purpose of chest compression is to move oxygenated blood or drugs to the coronary arteries in order to initiate cardiac recovery. Thus there is no point in starting chest compression before effective lung inflation has been established. Similarly, compressions are ineffective unless interposed by ventilation breaths of good quality. Therefore, the emphasis must be upon good-quality breaths, followed by effective compressions. Simultaneous delivery of compressions and breaths should be avoided, as the former will reduce the effectiveness of the breaths. It is usually only necessary to continue chest compressions for about 20–30 s before the heart responds with an increase in heart rate, so reassess after this period.

Once the heart rate is > 60 min[-1] and rising, chest compression can be discontinued. Maintain ventilations at 30 min[-1] until effective breathing or mechanical ventilation is established.

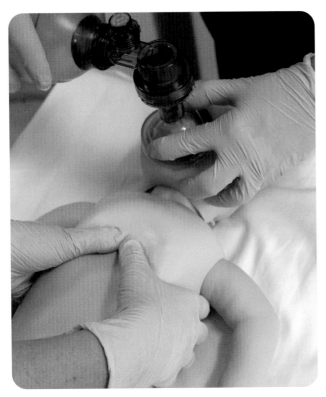

Figure 12.3 Chest compression on a newborn infant: Two thumb encircling technique

Drugs

If after adequate lung inflation and cardiac compression the heart rate has not responded, drug therapy should be considered. However, the most common reason for failure of the heart rate to respond is failure to achieve lung inflation, and there is no point in giving drugs unless the airway is open and the lungs have been inflated. Airway and breathing must be reassessed as adequate before proceeding to drug therapy. Venous access will be required via an umbilical venous line (or rarely through an intraosseus needle). The outcome is poor if drugs are required for resuscitation.

Adrenaline

Adrenaline increases coronary artery perfusion during resuscitation, enhancing oxygen delivery to the heart. In the presence of profound unresponsive bradycardia or circulatory standstill, 10 mcg kg^{-1} (0·1 mL kg^{-1} 1:10000) adrenaline may be given intravenously. Further doses of 10–30 mcg kg^{-1} (0·1–0·3 mL 1:10000) may be tried at 3–5 min intervals if there is no response. The tracheal route is not recommended.

Bicarbonate

Any baby who is in terminal apnoea will have a significant metabolic acidosis. Acidosis depresses cardiac function. Bicarbonate 1–2 mmol kg^{-1} (2–4 mL kg^{-1} of 4·2% solution) may be used to raise the pH and enhance the effects of oxygen and adrenaline.

Bicarbonate use remains controversial and it should only be used in the absence of discernible cardiac output

despite all resuscitative efforts or in profound and unresponsive bradycardia.

Glucose

Hypoglycaemia is a potential problem for all stressed or asphyxiated babies. It is treated using a slow bolus of 2.5 mL kg^{-1} of 10% glucose intravenously, and then providing a secure intravenous glucose infusion at a rate of 100 mL kg^{-1} day^{-1} of 10% glucose. BM stix are not reliable in neonates when reading < 5 mmol L^{-1}.

Fluid

Very occasionally hypovolaemia may be present because of known or suspected blood loss (antepartum haemorrhage, placenta or vasa praevia, unclamped cord) or it may be secondary to loss of vascular tone following asphyxia. Volume expansion, initially with 10 mL kg^{-1}, may be appropriate. 0.9% saline can be used; if blood loss is acute and severe, non-cross-matched O-negative blood should be given immediately. However, most newborn or neonatal resuscitations do not require fluid unless there has been known blood loss or septicaemic shock.

Response to resuscitation

The first indication of success will be an increase in heart rate. Recovery of respiratory drive may be delayed. Babies in terminal apnoea will tend to gasp first as they recover before starting normal respirations. Those who were in primary apnoea are likely to start with normal breaths, which may commence at any stage of resuscitation.

Tracheal intubation

Most babies can be resuscitated using a mask system. However, tracheal intubation, if it is performed, is especially useful in prolonged resuscitations, pre-term babies and meconium aspiration. It should be considered if mask ventilation has failed, although the most common reason for failure with mask ventilation is poor positioning of the head with consequent failure to open the airway or poor application of the mask resulting in a leak.

The technique of intubation is the same as for infants and is described in Chapter 4. A normal full-term newborn usually needs a 3·5 mm tracheal tube, but 4·0, 3·0 and 2·5 mm tubes should also be available.

Tracheal tube placement must be assessed visually during intubation and in most cases will be confirmed by a rapid response in heart rate on ventilating via the tracheal tube. End-tidal CO_2 detection will correctly identify most correctly sited tubes in the presence of any cardiac output. Detection of exhaled carbon dioxide should be used to confirm tracheal tube placement along with chest X-ray.

Special Cases

Pre-term babies

Unexpected deliveries outside delivery suites are more likely to be premature. Premature babies are more likely to get cold (higher surface area to mass ratio), and more likely to become hypoglycaemic (fewer glycogen stores). There are now several trials which support the use of plastic bags placed over babies of < 32 weeks' gestation or < 1000 g before drying in order to keep them warm. The babies should then be placed under a radiant heater.

The lungs of pre-term babies are more fragile than those of term babies and thus are much more susceptible to damage from over-distension. Therefore, it is appropriate to start with a lower inflation pressure of 20–25 cm H_2O but do not be afraid to increase this to 30 cm H_2O if there is no heart rate response.

It should be noted that very obvious chest wall movement in premature babies of < 28 weeks gestation may indicate excessive and potentially damaging tidal volumes.

Premature babies are more susceptible to the toxic effects of hyperoxia. Resuscitation is commenced using air (21%) to 30% oxygen and a pulse oximeter is used to monitor both heart rate and oxygen saturation in these babies from birth. At present, additional oxygen should not be given if the oxygen saturation from the right arm or wrist is above the values given in Table 12.2.

Actions in the event of poor initial response to resuscitation

1. Check airway and breathing.

2. Check for a technical fault.

    (a) Is mask ventilation effective? Observe movement.

    (b) Is the tracheal tube in the trachea? Auscultate both axillae, listen at the mouth for a large leak, and observe movement. Use an end-tidal CO_2 detector to ensure tracheal tube position.

    (c) Is the tracheal tube in the right bronchus? Auscultate both axillae and observe movement.

    (d) Is the tracheal tube blocked? If there is doubt about the position or patency of the tracheal tube re-place it. Use an end-tidal CO_2 detector.

    (e) Is a longer inflation time required?

    (f) If starting in air then increase the oxygen concentration. This is least likely to be a cause, although if monitoring saturations it could be a cause for slow increase.

3. Does the baby have a pneumothorax? This occurs spontaneously in up to 1% of newborns, but those needing action in the delivery unit are exceptionally rare. Auscultate the chest for asymmetry of breath sounds. A cold light source can be used to transilluminate the chest – a pneumothorax may show as a hyper-illuminating area.

4. Does the baby remain cyanosed despite breathing with a good heart rate? There may be a congenital heart

malformation, which may be duct-dependent or a persistent pulmonary hypertension.

5. Is there severe anaemia or hypovolaemia? In case of large blood loss, 10 mL^{-1} of O negative blood or a volume expander should be given.

Discontinuation of resuscitation

The outcome for a baby with no detectable cardiac output for more than 10 min is likely to be very poor. Stopping resuscitation early, or not starting resuscitation at all, may be appropriate in situations of extreme prematurity (< 23 weeks) or with birth weight of < 400 g.

Summary learning

- **Most babies need no more than drying, keeping warm and given to mother.**
- **The key to successful resuscitation at birth is lung inflation.**
- **Start resuscitation with air – only add oxygen if SpO$_2$ remains low despite good lung inflation and ventilation.**

My key take-home messages from this chapter

Further reading

Newborn Life Support Manual 2011, 2016, Resuscitation Council UK

European Resuscitation Council Guidelines for Resuscitation 2015 Section 7. Resuscitation and support of transition of babies at birth. Wyllie J, Bruinenberg J, Roehr CC, Rüdiger M, Trevisanuto D, Urlesberger B. Resuscitation 2015;95;249-263.

Part 7: Neonatal resuscitation2015 International Consensus on Cardiopulmonary Resuscitation and Emergency Cardiovascular Care Science with Treatment Recommendations. Jonathan Wyllie (Co-Chair), Jeffrey M. Perlman (Co-Chair), John Kattwinkel, Myra H. Wyckoff, Khalid Aziz, Ruth Guinsburg, Han-Suk Kim, Helen G. Liley, Lindsay Mildenhall, Wendy M. Simon, Edgardo Szyld, Masanori Tamura, Sithembiso Velaphi, on behalf of the Neonatal Resuscitation Chapter Collaborator Resuscitation 2015:95;e169-e201.

Ethical considerations in resuscitation

Contents

- **Ethical concepts and principles**
- **Do not attempt cardiopulmonary resuscitation (DNACPR)**
- **Presence of parents during resuscitation attempts**

Learning outcomes

To enable you to:

- **Understand the legal and ethical implications of 'duty of care' with regard to paediatric resuscitation**
- **Discuss the indications for not starting resuscitation and the implications of this decision**
- **Consider the relevant factors when deciding to discontinue a resuscitation attempt**

Ethical concepts and principles

Ethics is the field of study that attempts to understand human actions in a moral sense. Medical ethics is the study of the application of moral principles that guide the behaviour of healthcare professionals. Ethical principles are not immutable; they change over time and vary according to the social and cultural characteristics of the human populace.

Historically the ethics of medical practice was guided by the Hippocratic principle 'Do good and avoid harm' without any recognition of the patient's opinion. Now, the central role of the patient (or parents/guardians in the case of a child) in the decision-making process is recognised. In the current approach to medical ethics, four guiding principles are considered:

- Autonomy
- Beneficence
- Justice
- Non-maleficence.

Dignity and honesty are frequently added as essential elements.

Autonomy

Autonomy requires people to be allowed and helped to make their own informed decisions, rather than having decisions made for them. A person with capacity must be adequately informed about the matter to be decided and free from undue pressure in making their decision. Autonomy allows an informed person to make a choice, even if that choice is considered illogical or incorrect by others, including health professionals. As a child's sense of autonomy evolves, children have a right to have their opinion taken into account when decisions are being made that affect them directly. An inclusive approach of both parents and guardians as well as the child is fundamental to ensure that the parents/guardians have been correctly informed and that they fully understand the

EUROPEAN PAEDIATRIC
ADVANCED LIFE SUPPORT

clinical situation, the treatment plan and alternatives before making a treatment decision. If the patient is not competent, because of age or disturbance of mental capability, the parents/guardians must make the decision on his behalf. The patient has a right to confidentiality: the doctor must inform only the patient and those individuals he wishes to be informed; this may cause conflict particularly concerning sick adolescents. The only exception to this is in the event of serious criminal actions where not informing a relevant authority would seriously jeopardise public welfare.

Competence

There may be occasions where a parent is absent and a condition is not life-threatening so professionals feel they cannot treat a child without parental/guardian permission but there is a degree of urgency. It may be a young person can give consent to treatment without the parent's consent, even if under 16 years. The criteria which are used to determine if a young person under 16 years of age can give consent are known as the "Fraser guidelines". These guidelines originated n the area of contraception. The Mental Health capacity Act 2005 is the definitive legal document covering detailed issues concerning children's consent. All children aged 16 years and over are considered to have the capacity to consent to treatment unless there is evidence to the contrary.

The young person must understand the advice given and have sufficient maturity to consider the implications of what is involved. The child must be able to retain the information and comprehend the nature, purpose and consequences of the treatment (or lack of it),and be able to communicate their decision. An example might include a limb-threatening rather than life-threatening injury in a young teenager. The clinician must acknowledge that without the treatment, the young person's physical health may be at risk.

There may be occasions where the clinician disagrees with the parents. In a life-threatening situation the clinician may act in the best interests of the child. If there is time the case can go to court for a judicial decision. In this instance, it is advisable that the clinician contact his defence organisation.

If a competent child is refusing treatment then those with parental responsibility can consent to treatment if this is in the child's best interests.

Beneficence

All medical acts must be guided by the goal of achieving good for the patient whilst balancing benefit and risk. This principle requires that the patient is offered all available diagnostic procedures and potentially beneficial therapies.

Evidence-based clinical guidelines exist to assist decision-making. Increasingly, patients and guardians are involved as active partners in a personalised protocol or guideline development process, ensuring that patient's views and perspectives are captured in the guidance provided.

Justice

This requires spreading benefits and risks equally within a society to guarantee equal opportunities and a rational distribution of resources. There should be no discrimination purely on grounds of factors such as age, race, religion, socioeconomics or disability. Justice does not imply an entitlement to expect or demand CPR for everyone. In addition, medical practice must conform to civilian and criminal law.

Non-maleficence

The actions of healthcare professionals must not cause harm. Treatments that are harmful must be avoided. The balance between risks and benefits of a proposed treatment for a patient must be evaluated carefully. Only treatments that have demonstrated efficacy should be used but futility is difficult to define in a way that is precise, prospective and applies to the majority of cases.

Ethical aspects of paediatric life support

Cardiorespiratory arrest and other clinical emergencies can be unpredictable. There may not have been an opportunity to discuss treatment options with the child and/or parents/guardian before the event. In these circumstances, the principle of a child's autonomy is difficult to apply and healthcare professionals must make the decisions about resuscitation. In these situations, consent for life-saving interventions is presumed.

For children, information must be given to the parents/guardians, unless the nature of the emergency does not allow for this. If the parents/guardians are present, they can be given information as the resuscitation takes place; if they are not, the circumstances must be carefully documented in the child's medical records. In some cases, there may be conflicts of interest between parents, or they may refuse appropriate and effective treatment because of religious or other beliefs. If this occurs, the doctor must make a decision that protects the best interests of the child and he should request both legal advice and advice of colleagues. Carefully detailed documentation including the reasons for the decision is required.

Ethics and cardiorespiratory resuscitation

When to start resuscitation

Life support should be started in the following circumstances unless a valid DNACPR decision exists:

- Sudden and unexpected cardiorespiratory arrest.

- Recent cardiorespiratory arrest. However, if there is a delay in initiating resuscitation following cardiorespiratory arrest of more than 30 min, or if there are signs of established biological death, life support should not be started (with the exception of drowning and/or hypothermia).

- Potentially reversible causes precipitate the cardiorespiratory arrest.

- Non-terminal illness. Resuscitation is not indicated if the cardiorespiratory arrest is the final natural end event in a process of dying after all available treatment options have been exhausted. The right to die with suitable dignity must be respected.

- A DNACPR decision does not exist.

- There is no risk to the rescuer.

- There are potential/actual safe-guarding issues. Legal as well as ethical implications of a child's care need to be considered. All clothes should be kept in marked bags for forensic purposes.

When to stop resuscitation

Resuscitation should be terminated when:

- There are signs of established biological death.

- The rescuer is too exhausted to continue or is in danger.

- Other victims who have a greater chance of survival require simultaneous life support but there are insufficient numbers of people to carry out resuscitation.

- A DNACPR decision exists.

- In newborn babies, after 10 min of optimal resuscitation, discontinuation may be justified if there are no signs of life.

- ***Consider and discuss the option of discontinuing resuscitation*** if life support has been continued for at least 20–30 min without evidence of a return of spontaneous circulation (other factors should also be considered such as cause, age, presenting rhythm).

However, resuscitation should be continued:

  - in hypothermic children

  - in cases of poisoning

  - in persistent ventricular fibrillation

  - when cardiorespiratory arrest occurs in children with invasive monitoring in place (whereby coronary perfusion pressure can be continuously assessed, ensuring that an adequate cardiac output can be generated to perfuse vital organs)

  - when the team considers (based on specific circumstances) that resuscitation efforts must be maintained.

Organ donation

International consensus is that brain stem death is equivalent to the death of the person. This is recognised under UK law but not always in other countries. When brain stem death has occurred, the only rationale for maintaining cardiorespiratory function is to allow further investigations, discussions and permissions for organ donation. In these circumstances, if cardiac activity stops, resuscitation would be inappropriate.

Donation of an organ should be requested in the event of brain stem death, or cardiac valve or other tissue donation can be considered in the event of cardiac death. The approach to the family of the potential organ donor must be sensitive and respectful. Frequently this request is accepted, usually 'to help other children'. The donation should not impair the bereavement process of the child's family. Sometimes parents change their mind many hours after a child's death when some organs may still be useful (e.g. corneas). Seek specialist advice as soon as possible.

Contraindications to organ donation are:

- cancers, except for certain non-metastatic brain tumours

- some metabolic diseases

- specific infections

- caution if history of intravenous drug addiction; further investigations may be indicated.

Making decisions about CPR

When someone is dying from an irreversible cause, CPR is unlikely to work but can subject them to an undignified death, or even cause suffering and prolong the process of dying. Prolonging life at all costs is not an appropriate goal of medicine.

If a child is at risk of death or sudden cardiac arrest, consider in advance whether or not CPR could help them and whether they or their parents or guardians would want CPR. Whenever possible, make advance plans as shared decisions with parents, guardians and or patients as part of a wider consideration of other care and realistic treatments that may or may not be appropriate for each child. Avoid focusing specifically on cardiac arrest or CPR or completing a form. Start by establishing a shared understanding of the patient's condition and likely future developments. Explore the child and parents' or guardians' priorities and preferences for their child's future care. Then discuss what types of care and realistic treatment will help them to achieve their goals of care, and whether or not they would want them, and explain relevant treatments that would not work or could do harm. Discuss CPR within this context of the broader treatment options, which might include, for example, emergency admission to hospital, various types of organ support such as ventilation, or antibiotics for life-threatening infection. Effective communication is essential to ensure that decisions about treatments such as CPR are made well and understood clearly by all those involved. The courts have made clear that there should be a presumption in favour of involving patients and or parents and families in discussions about whether or not CPR will be attempted. This upholds the principle of autonomy and the provisions of the Human Rights Act (1998).

Recording parents', guardians' or a child's wishes about these other aspects of the child's care and treatment, alongside recommendations about CPR, can help to guide immediate decision-making by health or care professionals faced with helping that person (who they may not have met before) in an emergency.

Requirements for effective communication include providing information in a format that the parents, guardians and or child can understand, and checking that they have understood it. They may need time and more than one discussion before they can reach a shared decision that they are comfortable with. They should be offered opportunities for further discussion and be made aware that they may change their decision if they wish to.

It is not necessary to discuss CPR with parents or guardians if there is no reason to expect the child to suffer cardiac arrest or die. However, if any parent, guardian or child wants to discuss CPR they must be given full opportunity to do so.

Make sure that you are familiar with the approach and policy that is used in your health and care community or organisation. Various forms have been developed in different places to record people's treatment decisions in advance. The RC (UK) favours the use of a standard document that is used and accepted by all health and care provider organisations, so that it is effective across geographical and organisational boundaries. It supports use of the ReSPECT process and form: www.respectprocess.org.uk.

In addition, all health and care professionals must practise within the law. Laws relevant to CPR, including those on matters relating to capacity and consent, vary from nation to nation, both outside and within the UK. Detailed guidance, *Decisions relating to cardiopulmonary resuscitation*, has been published by the British Medical Association (BMA), Resuscitation Council (UK) (RC (UK)) and Royal College of Nursing (RCN). It includes guidance on ethical and legal aspects of decisions about CPR, but the ethical and legal principles that underpin this guidance apply equally to the broader planning approach taken by the ReSPECT process and other treatment escalation plans. As an EPALS provider you should read and be familiar with that guidance, and be familiar with relevant aspects of the law in the nation where you live and work.

Presence of parents during resuscitation

Parents of children suffering from chronic diseases may be used to assisting with medical procedures and are often present during the resuscitation of their children.

The majority of parents would like to be present during resuscitation. Parents witnessing their child's resuscitation can see that everything possible has been attempted. Families who are present at their child's death show less anxiety and depression, better adjustment and an improved grieving process when assessed several months later.

The opportunity to be present during resuscitation should be offered to parents. If they decide to stay, a dedicated member of the team must be assigned to explain the process to them in an empathetic manner, thereby ensuring that the parents do not interfere with resuscitation. When appropriate, physical contact with the child should be allowed and, wherever possible, the parents should be permitted to be with their dying child in the final moments.

The resuscitation team leader will decide when to stop resuscitation. This must be expressed to the parents with sensitivity and understanding.

Informing parents

When a child dies, it is the resuscitation team leader's duty to inform the parents. This is always a difficult task, particularly if the parents were not present at the resuscitation and the suddenness of an event may make it difficult for the team leader to understand family dynamics and predict a response to bad news.

The following four principles may ease the process, preparation, communication, planning and follow-up:

- Select an appropriate environment (with assured privacy).

- The medical attitude must be professional, with a simple and clear explanation of the facts, but at the same time it should be compassionate and the emotional needs of the parents must be recognised. It is important to take a few moments to prepare what the team leader will say.

- Establish with certainty who the family members are, and their relationship to the child.

- Explain with clarity that their child is dead (use the word "dead" specifically). Information should be given with empathy, compassion and sympathy. The details of the circumstances should be given clearly. Use the child's first name and avoid 'empty introductory sentences' (he came in with.. and we tried.. but eventually we failed and..) that postpone saying the only thing parents are waiting to hear ('alive or dead').

- Encourage the parents to see and stay with their child. They should be encouraged to touch and hold their child.

- Explain the necessity of a post-mortem examination (if applicable), particularly in cases of sudden, unexplained or accidental death. Inform the parents that the police and the coroner are routinely informed if the child's death fits these circumstances and consider other safe guarding issues.

- Permission for post-mortem studies may be discussed with the parents where this may help better understanding of aspects of the child's condition or mode of death.

- Ask the parents about any religious requirements.

- Do not guess at the diagnosis but explain that the pathologist will try to ascertain the cause of death. Explain that all children's deaths in England and Wales are reviewed by Child Death Overview panels (part of local Sagfeguarding Children's Board) and it is normal in unexpected deaths that a rapid response team is convened to co-ordinate investigations.

- Make an appointment for further discussion and information.

Verify

- name and address of parents
- date of birth of the deceased child
- arrival time in the emergency department (if relevant)
- time of death.

Inform

- paediatrician or general practitioner, giving the address where the parents are going and their contact details

- health visitor for children < 5 years or school nurse for children > 5 years

- social worker

- persons that the parents wish to be informed

- document this information in the child's notes and ensure their safe keeping.

Summary learning

- **Ethics attempts to understand human actions in a moral sense.**
- **In current medical ethics, the four guiding principles are: autonomy, beneficence, non-maleficence and justice.**
- **Information must be given to the child as appropriate and to the parents/guardians.**
- **The majority of parents would like to be present during resuscitation.**
- **If the child dies, parents being present during resuscitation helps their grieving process.**

My key take-home messages from this chapter

Further reading

Beckman AW, Sloan BK, Moore GP et al. Should parents be present during emergency department procedures on children, and who should make that decision? A survey of emergency physician and nurse attitudes. Acad Emerg Med 2002; 9: 154-8.

British Medical Association, Resuscitation Council (UK) and Royal College of Nursing. Decisions relating to cardiopulmonary resuscitation. 2007. www.resus.org.uk

Boie ET, Moore GP, Brummett C, Nelson DR. Do parents want to be present during invasive procedures performed on their children in the emergency department? A survey of 400 parents. Ann Emerg Med 1999; 34: 70-4.

Horisberger T, Fischer JE, Fanconi S. One-year survival and neurological outcome after pediatric cardiopulmonary resuscitation. Int Care Med 2002; 28: 365-8.

Powers KS, Rubenstein JS. Family presence during invasive procedures in the pediatric intensive care unit: a prospective study. Arch Pediatr Adoles Med 1999; 153: 955-8.

Meyers TA, Eichhorn DJ, Guzzetta CE et al. Family presence during invasive procedures and resuscitation. Am J Nurs 2000; 100: 32-42.

Sacchetti A, Lichenstein R, Carraccio CA, Harris RH. Family member presence during pediatric emergency department procedures. Pediatr Emerg Care 1996;12: 268-71.

Robinson SM, Mackenzie-Ross S, Campbell Hewson GL, Egleston CV, Prevost AT. Psychological effect of witnessed resuscitation on bereaved relatives (comment). Lancet 1998; 352: 614-7.

Sharp MC, Strauss RP, Lorch RC. Communicating medical bad news: parents' experiences and preferences. J Pediatr 1992; 121: 539-46.

Taylor N, Bonilla L, Silver P, Sagy M. Pediatric procedure: do parents want to be present? Crit Care Med 1996; 24: A131.

Tsai E. Should family members be present during cardiopulmonary resuscitation? N Engl J Med 2002; 346: 1019-21.

Woolley H, Stein A, Forest GC et al. Imparting the diagnosis of life threatening illness in children. BMJ 1989; 298: 1623-6.

Youngblut JM, Shiao SYP. Child and family reactions during and after pediatric ICU hospitalization: a pilot study. Heart Lung 1993; 22: 46-54.

I. Barata, J. LaMantia, D. Riccardi, et al: A Prospective Study of Emergency Medicine Residents' Attitudes toward Family Presence during Pediatric Procedures. . The Internet Journal of Emergency Medicine. 2007; 3:number 2.

L.Nibert, D.Ondrejka Family presence during pediatric resuscitation: An integrative review for evidence-based practice Journal of Pediatric Nursing 2005; Volume 20: Issue 2,145-147.

http://www.dca.gov.uk/menincap/legis.htm

SCOPE package for training in delivering bad news. http://www.rcn.org.uk/__data/assets/pdf_file/0006/545289/004471.pdf. accessed 23 Sept2015

Working together to safeguard children. http://www.workingtogetheronline.co.uk/chapters/chapter_five.html accessed 23 Sept 2015

Organ donation information for UK, Scotland, Wales, Northern Ireland
https://www.organdonation.nhs.uk/about-donation/what-can-i-donate/
https://www.organdonationscotland.org/
http://organdonationwales.org/?skip=1&lang=en
https://www.organdonationni.info/

www.respectprocess.org.uk

EPALS

140

Non-technical skills in resuscitation

Contents

- **Non-technical skills**
- **Situational awareness**
- **Decision making**
- **Team working including leadership**
- **Task management**
- **Resuscitation audit**

Learning outcomes

To enable you to:

- **Understand the role of non-technical skills in resuscitation**
- **Discuss the roles of team leader and team member**
- **Appreciate the importance of communication tools such as SBAR and RSVP for both summoning help and for handover**

Non-technical skills

Paediatric resuscitation is particularly emotive and stressful and sometimes highly time critical. Outcomes can be improved by forward planning and practising teamwork skills and communication. The resuscitation team may take the form of a traditional cardiac arrest team, which is called only when cardiorespiratory arrest is recognised. However, many hospitals now have medical emergency teams who can manage sick children at risk of cardiorespiratory arrest and facilitate effective treatment thereby preventing it. The term 'resuscitation team' in this manual reflects the range of response teams.

On-call teams should meet before shift changes/handovers, introduce each other and decide on role allocation. This 'huddle' prepares the team, maximises the team's ability to work closely and focus on the best care for the patient. After an emergency it is equally important to reflect on and scrutinise every aspect of the resuscitation from response times through to team actions and communication in order to identify areas for improvement.

Traditionally, advanced life support courses have focused mainly on skills: chest compressions, defibrillation, rhythm recognition and vascular access and the knowledge required to deliver optimal care. There is now a paradigm shift stressing the importance of many non-technical skills including communication, leadership, mutual support from team members, task distribution and situational awareness, leading to better decision making.

Deficiencies in the requisite non-technical skills are a common cause of adverse incidents which studies have shown impact markedly on the outcome of the resuscitation. Such deficiencies include:

EUROPEAN PAEDIATRIC
ADVANCED LIFE SUPPORT

- errors in calling the resuscitation team

- failure to start CPR

- late or non-arrival of personnel

- lack of organised cooperation in the team

- lack of leadership

- poor communication.

Non-technical skills describe communication, situational awareness, decision-making, team working including leadership and task management.

Communication

- Lack of clear and concise communication problems are factors in up to 80% of adverse incidents or near-miss reports in hospitals.

- Communication is vital in every stage of managing a sick child: summoning help, preparing for the resuscitation, during the resuscitation and organising the post-resuscitation care.

- The use of either the SBAR (Situation, Background, Assessment, Recommendation) or RSVP (Reason, Story, Vital signs, Plan) tool enables effective, timely communication between individuals from different clinical backgrounds and hierarchies and this can apply to both summoning help and performing a handover. When individuals are faced with a deteriorating patient they should request help by presenting a succinct summary to a senior colleague. The SBAR and RSVP systems are validated tools for this purpose (Table 14.1). Clear unambiguous communication ensures that help arrives, information is handed over in a clear fashion, likely to be understood quickly and facilitates incorporation of a new team leader or team member.

Example of good communication:

A nurse finding a patient collapsed with no breathing or pulse asks her colleague to call the resuscitation team.

"John, this child is in cardiorespiratory arrest, please dial 2222 and call the resuscitation team. Come back immediately with BMV when you have made the call".

Preparation

Responsibilities of a team leader:

Pre-planning during the 'huddle' helps the team identify a team leader (TL) who allocates tasks to different team members (TM) according to skill mix, identifying any immediate need for further senior help. Depending upon the number of team members the TL will assign tasks:

- airway and ventilation tasks TM1

- pulse check and chest compressions TM2 (alternate

TM2 and TM5 for chest compressions and recording/drug preparation)

- attaching monitoring, pads and/or defibrillating as indicated TM3

- gaining IO/IV access, preparing and delivering drugs TM4

- recording events, drug preparation TM5 (TM2).

Relatives can be looked after by another member of staff (e.g. TM6). This should not be the most junior member of staff as parents need careful explanation of the events .

After two minutes rescuers doing chest compressions become less effective so this task should be rotated with other team members. In the example above TM2 is alternated with TM5 but this is just a suggestion, the TL can ask other team members to alternate if more appropriate. Ideally this change should be pre-planned and communicated to the rest of the team. The team should also focus on delivery of high quality CPR and use of feedback devices is recommended to guide this.

Clinical staff who participate as members of the resuscitation team must be up to date with advanced skills in paediatric life support, including resuscitation algorithms. They must be familiar and practiced with local equipment such as defibrillator, IO needles and auto-injectors.

It is also important that resuscitation teams practice skills together to try to avoid error. This may involve high and low-fidelity scenarios on courses such as EPALS and involve on-site mock clinical emergency team calls.

Management of the resuscitation event

Preparation can help, if there is time, by writing up predicted airway, fluid and drug requirements. Remember, exact weight estimation is not necessary as most resuscitation drugs are based on lean weight.

During the resuscitation event the team leader:

- addresses clear commands directly to individuals to retain focus

- uses "closed loop" techniques to ensure tasks have been completed

- asks individuals in turn to report findings from airway, breathing and circulation assessments, addressing problems as they are found.

Situational awareness

This can be described as an individual's awareness of the environment at any one moment and their ability to respond. How individuals react may impact on future events, this becomes particularly important when many events are happening simultaneously (e.g. at a cardiorespiratory arrest).

SBAR	RSVP	Content	Example
SITUATION	**R**EASON	• Introduce yourself and check you are speaking to the correct person • Identify the patient you are calling about (who and where) • Say what you think the current problem is, or appears to be • State what you need advice about • Useful phrases: - The problem appears to be cardiac/respiratory/neurological/sepsis - I'm not sure what the problem is but the patient is deteriorating - The patient is unstable, getting worse and I need help	• Hi, I'm Dr Smith the paediatric F2 • I am calling about Sam Brown on the paediatric ward who I think has a severe pneumonia and is septic • He has an oxygen saturation of 90% despite high-flow oxygen and I am very worried about him
BACKGROUND	**S**TORY	• Background information about the patient • Reason for admission • Relevant past medical history	• He is 6 years old and previously fit and well • He has had fever and a cough for 2 days • He was admitted yesterday
ASSESSMENT	**V**ITAL SIGNS	• Include specific observations and vital sign values based on ABCDE approach • Airway • Breathing • Circulation • Disability • Exposure • The early warning score is...	• He looks very unwell and is tiring • Airway – he can say a few words • Breathing – his respiratory rate is 34, he has widespread wheeze in both lung fields and has bronchial breathing on the left side. His oxygen saturation is 90% on high-flow oxygen. I am getting a blood gas and chest X-ray • Circulation – his pulse is 180, his blood pressure is 90/60 • Disability – he is drowsy and is clinging onto his mum • Exposure – he has no rashes
RECOMMENDATION	**P**LAN	• State explicitly what you want the person you are calling to do • What by when? • Useful phrases: - I am going to start the following treatment; is there anything else you can suggest? - I am going to do the following investigations; is there anything else you can suggest? - If they do not improve; when would you like to be called? - I don't think I can do any more; I would like you to see the patient urgently	• He is only on oral antibiotics so I am starting an IV • I need help – please can you come and see him straight away?

Table 14.1 SBAR and RSVP communication tools

Poor decisions will be made if too much information is provided at the same time, especially if this is coupled with a lack of situational awareness (e.g. long pauses in CPR are unnoticed). At a cardiorespiratory arrest, all those participating will have varying degrees of situational awareness which may be appropriate as they focus on their given tasks. In a well-functioning team, the team leader ensures all members will have a common understanding of current events, or shared situational awareness. This may be done by the team leader intermittently succinctly summing-up the situation, actions taken so far and planned actions giving time for team members to provide any additional information or comment as appropriate. It is important that only the relevant information is shared.

Important situational awareness factors include:

- consideration of the location of the arrest, which can give clues to the cause

- obtaining information from staff about the events leading up to the arrest

- confirmation of the diagnosis if known or keeping track of tests ordered

- noting actions already initiated (e.g. chest compressions)

- checking that a monitor been attached and interpreting the rhythm

- gathering information from team members

- implementing any immediate necessary action and consideration of the likely impact of interventions

- determining the immediate needs

- not losing awareness of the overall situation when encountering difficult to overcome problems.

Decision making

This is defined as the cognitive process of choosing a specific course of action from several alternatives. At a cardiorespiratory arrest, decision making usually falls to the team leader who may be a nurse or doctor. The leader needs to establish their role quickly if not pre-planned, and assimilate information from those present to determine appropriate interventions. Typical decisions made include:

- confirmation of cardiorespiratory arrest and continuation of CPR

- attaching a monitor and assessing the rhythm

- delivering a shock if indicated

- considering the likely causes of the cardiac arrest.

Team working, including team leadership

A team is a group of people collaborating, cooperating and coordinating their activities towards a common goal. Team leadership can be taught, observed and practised. Team membership can be improved by rehearsal, reflection and coaching producing effective teams which lead them to perform well together.

Team leadership

The management of a sick child requires a team leader who communicates clearly providing guidance, direction, instruction and an overall update to the team members. Team leaders are facilitators, leading by example and integrity, and need experience, not simply seniority. Team leadership is achieved as a process, thereby it can become available to everyone with training and it is not restricted to those with leadership traits. There are several factors recognisable in good team leaders:

- Ideally, the team leader knows everyone in the team by name and knows their capability.

- Accepts the leadership role and announces it early preferably at start of shift huddle so it is clear who is leading the team; this is very important as many people are reluctant to 'step up' and precious time is lost. The leader does need to be assertive and authoritative when appropriate and both knowledgeable and credible to influence the team through role modelling and professionalism.

- Is able to delegate tasks appropriately.

- The team leader should update the team, keeping them in the 'big picture' and should help include late additions to the team. This enables team members to offer constructive ideas/solutions or to challenge possible erroneous decisions. A leader will follow current resuscitation guidelines or explain the reasoning for any significant deviation from standard protocols. If a leader is unsure of a diagnosis or how to proceed then he or she should consult with the team or call for senior advice and assistance as appropriate.

- Remains calm and keeps everyone focused and controls distractions.

- Is a good communicator – not just good at giving instructions, also a good listener and decisive in action. A good leader also shows tolerance towards hesitancy or nervousness in the emergency setting, showing empathy towards the whole team.

- Allow the team autonomy if their skills are adequate (e.g. the anaesthetist may be delegated to be responsible for the airway management so 'leadership' of the airway is the anaesthetist's responsibility. When the airway is secured the anaesthetist should inform the team leader.

- Use the two-minute periods of chest compressions to prioritise and plan tasks and safety aspects of the resuscitation attempt with the team. If a case is particularly complex it may be necessary for the leadership style to change from facilitative to directive in order to drive the speed of treatment in the time critical situation.

- The team leader needs to watch for fatigue, stress and distress amongst the team and manage conflict.

- At the end of the resuscitation attempt, the leader should thank the team and ensure that staff and relatives are being supported and kept fully informed. Complete all documentation and ensure an adequate handover by planned communication with experts either by telephone or in person.

- Debriefing the team, and untoward incidents reported, particularly equipment or system failures (see below). Audit forms should be completed and this may be carried out by the leader or delegated as appropriate.

Team membership

Wherever possible, the duty team should meet at the beginning of their period on duty to form a 'huddle' as previously described. Any patients who have been identified as 'at risk' during the previous duty period should be reviewed.

Every effort should be made to enable the team members to meet at the end of their duty to debrief (Figure 14.1), (e.g. to discuss what went well and what could be improved). It may also be possible to carry out a formal handover to the incoming team.

Teamwork is one of the most important non-technical skills that contribute to successful management of critical situations. In a team, the members usually have complementary skills and can coordinate their efforts to work synergistically. There are several characteristics of a good resuscitation team member:

- Competence – has the skills required at a cardiorespiratory arrest and performs them to the best of their ability.

- Commitment – the team has a common goal, the best outcome for the patient.

- Communication – open, indicating their findings and actions taken.

Communication

Communication can be a challenge. Team leaders and team members should be considerate in their phraseology; in this way a leader can be challenged without raising stress levels for both the leader and team member.

Examples:

" I wonder if we should consider the use ...."

" I think we could try........"

" Should we get extra expert help now..?"

" I am happy to lead if you would appreciate the help....."

A good team member:

- listens carefully to briefings and instructions from the team leader

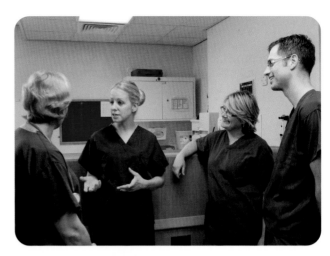

Figure 14.1 Team debrief

- is supportive and facilitative – allows others to achieve their best

- is accountable – for their own and the team's actions and recognises when help is needed

- may be creative, suggesting different ways of interpreting the situation

- participates in providing feedback

- helps the team to maintain situational awareness.

Task management

The many decisions to be made usually fall to the team leader who will assimilate information from the team members, personal observation and will use this to determine appropriate interventions. Typical decisions made include:

- planning and briefing the team, if feasible prior to the arrival of the patient

- sharing the initial plan and delegation of tasks to the team

- diagnosis of the cardiorespiratory arrest rhythm;

- choice of shock energy to be used for defibrillation;

- likely reversible causes of the cardiorespiratory arrest;

- decision making regarding how long to continue resuscitation

- to ensure that decisions have been implemented

- identification of resources required.

Post-resuscitation care

Resuscitation does not stop with return of spontaneous circulation (ROSC). Handing the patient over to another colleague or department, or to a different hospital all require good communication and the SBAR or RSVP tool can provide a framework for information sharing at this stage (Chapter 9).

High quality care

The Institute of Medicine defines that quality care is safe, effective, patient-centred, timely, efficient and equitable. Hospitals, resuscitation teams and EPALS providers should ensure they deliver these aspects of quality to improve the care of the deteriorating child and children in cardiorespiratory arrest. Two aspects of this are safety incident reporting (also called adverse or critical incident reporting) and collecting good quality data.

Safety incident reporting

Hospitals now report patient safety incidents to the NHS Commissioning Board Special Health Authority, which ensures patient safety is at the heart of the NHS, previously the domain of the National Patient Safety Agency (NPSA). A patient safety incident is defined as 'any unintended or unexpected incident that could have harmed or did lead to harm for one or more patients being cared for by the National Health Service (NHS). A review of NPSA safety incidents relating to cardiorespiratory arrest and patient deterioration by the Resuscitation Council (UK) shows that the most common reported incidents are associated with equipment problems, communication, delays in the resuscitation team attending and failure to escalate treatment.

Audit and outcome after cardiac arrest

Most modern defibrillators allow the cardiorespiratory arrest management to be downloaded with a time-line of different rhythms and actions taken in terms of defibrillation, cardioversion and cardiopulmonary resuscitation; it also allows quality of CPR delivered to be reviewed when a feedback device has been used. Locally, this useful information can help teams use reflection and feedback to improve future performance especially in terms of adherence to resuscitation guidelines, the percentage of time CPR has been performed and 'hands-off' time.

National audit of resuscitation processes and outcomes provides information about whether interventions and changes made to resuscitation guidelines improve patient care. New interventions that improve survival rate even marginally are important because of the many victims of cardiorespiratory arrest each year. Local hospitals or healthcare systems are unlikely to have sufficient patients to identify these effects or eliminate confounders. Therefore resuscitation outcome and processes should be reported in a standard manner to allow comparison between different areas of practice. The internationally agreed Utstein template is a standardised system of reporting that allows the comparison of resuscitation data across different countries and healthcare systems. This facilitates the use of large national and multi-national databases to evaluate the impact of new drugs or techniques.

In the UK, the National Cardiac Arrest Audit (NCAA) is an ongoing, national, comparative outcome audit of in-hospital cardiac arrests. It is a joint initiative between the Resuscitation Council (UK) and the Intensive Care National Audit & Research Centre (ICNARC) and is open to all acute hospitals in the UK and Ireland. The audit monitors and reports on the incidence of, and outcome from, in-hospital cardiorespiratory arrest in order to inform practice and policy. It aims to identify and foster improvements in the prevention, care delivery and outcomes from cardiorespiratory arrest. Data are collected according to standardised definitions and entered onto the NCAA secure web-based system. Once data are validated, hospitals are provided with activity reports and comparative reports, allowing a comparison of to be made not only within, but also between, hospitals locally, nationally and internationally. Furthermore it also enables the effects of introducing changes to guidelines, new drugs, new techniques etc to be monitored that would not be possible on a hospital-by-hospital basis.

Table 14.2 Outcomes following in-hospital cardiac arrest (UK) for children in participating hospitals 2015-2017 NCAA data. Total number Cardiac arrests = 1022

	VF/pVT	Asystole	PEA
% of arrests*	4.1%	23.9%	30.7%
% ROSC > 20 mins	74%	37%	66%
% Hospital discharge	72%	25%	47%
Overall survival to hospital discharge	51.1%		

*Remainder cardiac arrests bradycardia or other.

Summary learning

- **Non-technical skills are important during resuscitation.**
- **Use SBAR or RSVP for effective communication.**
- **Report safety incidents and collect cardiac arrest data to help improve patient care.**

My key take-home messages from this chapter

Further reading

Abella B, Edelson DP,Kim S, Retzer E, Myklebust H et al. CPR quality improvement during in-hospital cardiac arrest using a real-time audiovisual feedback system Resuscitation . 2007;73,1,54-61.

Andersen PO, Maaløe R, Andersen HR. Critical Incidents related to cardiac arrests reported to the Danish Safety Database. Resuscitation 2010;81,312-316.

Brand SI, Slee KM, Chang Yu-Hui, Cheng Meng-Ru, Lipinski CA et al. Team strategies and tools to enhance performance and safety training: The Effect of Training on both nursing staff perceptions regarding physician behaviours and patient satisfaction scores in the ED. Journal of Hospital Administration. 2015;4,48-53.

De Meester K, Verspuy M, Monsieurs K, Von Bogaert P. SBA improves nurse-physician communication and reduces unexpected deathe: A per and post intervention study. Resuscitation; 2013,84,1192-1196.

Flin R, O'Connor P, Crichton M. Safety at the Sharp End: a Guide to Non-Technical Skills. Aldershot: Ashgate, 2008.

Nolan JP et al. Incidence and outcome of in-hospital cardiac arrest in the UK NCAA. Resuscitation;2014;85,987-992.

Ornato JP, Peberdy MA et al. Impact of resuscitation system errors on survivors from in-hospital cardiac arrest. Resuscitation; 2012,83(1),63-69.

AGE	WEIGHT kg	ADRENALINE 1:10,000 · 10 mcg kg⁻¹ · IV, IO	FLUID BOLUS 0.9% Saline · 20 mL kg⁻¹ · IV, IO · Consider warmed fluids	GLUCOSE 10% · 2 mL kg⁻¹ · IV, IO · For known hypoglycaemia / Recheck glucose after dose And repeat as required	SODIUM BICARBONATE 4.2% · 1 mmol kg⁻¹ · IV, IO	SODIUM BICARBONATE 8.4% · 1 mmol kg⁻¹ · IV, IO	TRACHEAL TUBE UNCUFFED ID mm	TRACHEAL TUBE CUFFED ID mm (Monitor cuff pressure)	DEFIBRILLATION 4 joules kg⁻¹ · Trans-thoracic · Monophasic or biphasic · Manual
		mL	mL	mL	mL	mL	ID mm	ID mm	
<1 month	3.5	0.35	70	7	7	-	3.0	-	20
1 month	4	0.4	80	8	8	-	3.0 - 3.5	3.0	20
3 months	5	0.5	100	10	10	-	3.5	3.0	20
6 months	7	0.7	140	14	-	7	3.5	3.0	30
1 year	10	1.0	200	20	-	10	4.0	3.5	40
2 years	12	1.2	240	24	-	12	4.5	4.0	50
3 years	14	1.4	280	28	-	14	4.5 - 5.0	4.0 - 4.5	60
4 years	16	1.6	320	32	-	16	5.0	4.5	60
5 years	18	1.8	360	36	-	18	5.0 - 5.5	4.5 - 5.0	70
6 years	20	2.0	400	40	-	20	5.5	5.0	80
7 years	23	2.3	460	46	-	23	5.5 - 6.0	5.0 - 5.5	100
8 years	26	2.6	500	50	-	26	-	6.0 - 6.5	100
10 years	30	3.0	500	50	-	30	-	7.0	120
12 years	38	3.8	500	50	-	38	-	7 - 7.5	120
14 years	40	4.0	500	50	-	40	-	7 - 8	120 - 150
Adolescent	50kg	5.0	500	50	-	50	-	7 - 8	120 - 150
Adult	70kg	10.0	500	50	-	50	-	7 - 8	120 - 150

Cardioversion — Synchronised Shock – 1.0 joules kg⁻¹ escalating to 2.0 joules kg⁻¹ if unsuccessful.

Amiodarone — 5 mg kg⁻¹ IV or IO bolus in arrest (0.1 mL kg⁻¹ of 150 mg in 3 mL) after 3rd and 5th shocks. Flush line with 0.9% saline or 5% glucose.

Atropine — 20 mcg kg⁻¹, maximum dose 600 mcg.

Calcium chloride 10% — 0.2 mL kg⁻¹ for hypocalcaemia hyperkalaemia.

Lorazepam — 100 mcg kg⁻¹ IV or IO for treatment of seizures. Can be repeated after 10 min. Maximum single dose 4mg.

Adenosine — 100 mcg kg⁻¹ IV or IO for treatment of SVT. Second dose may be doubled requires large saline flush and ECG monitoring.

Anaphylaxis — Adrenaline 1:1000 **intramuscularly** (<6 yrs 150 mcg [0.15 mL], 6-12 yrs 300 mcg [0.3 mL], >12 yrs 500 mcg [0.5mL]) can be repeated after five min. (**OR** titrate boluses of 1 mcg kg⁻¹ IV **ONLY** if familiar with giving IV adrenaline).

Weights averaged on lean body mass from 50th centile weights for males and females. Drug doses based on Resuscitation Council (UK) Guidelines 2015 recommendations.
Recommendations for tracheal tubes are based on full term neonates.
For newborns glucose at 2.5mL kg⁻¹ is recommended.

EPALS

Useful links

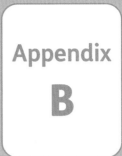

www.resus.org.uk	**Resuscitation Council (UK)**
www.erc.edu	**European Resuscitation Council**
www.ilcor.org	**International Liaison Committee on Resuscitation**
www.americanheart.org	**American Heart Association**
www.nice.org.uk	**The National Institute for Health and Care Excellence (NICE)**
www.rcpch.ac.uk	**Royal College of Paediatrics and Child Health**
www.bhf.org.uk	**British Heart Foundation**
www.ics.ac.uk	**Intensive Care Society**
www.aagbi.org	**Association of Anaesthetists of Great Britain and Ireland**
www.bestbets.org	**Best evidence topics in emergency medicine**
www.bcs.com	**British Cardiac Society**
www.escardio.org	**European Society of Cardiology**
www.esicm.org	**European Society of Intensive Care Medicine**

 Resuscitation Guidelines   **Resuscitation Council (UK) courses**

 iResus app – easy access to the Resuscitation Guidelines

 Lifesaver app – a new way to learn CPR

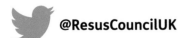 **@ResusCouncilUK**   **Resuscitation Council UK**   **ResusCouncilUK**